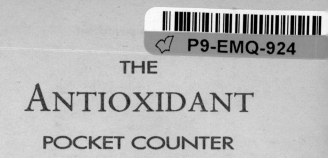

THE
ANTIOXIDANT
POCKET COUNTER

THE
ANTIOXIDANT
POCKET COUNTER

A Guide
to the Essential Nutrients
That Help Fight Cancer
and Heart Disease

Gail L. Becker, R.D.

Introduction by

Gladys Block, Ph.D.

TIMES 𝕋 BOOKS

RANDOM HOUSE

Library of Congress Cataloging-in-Publication Data

Becker, Gail L.
    The antioxidant pocket counter : a guide to the essential
nutrients that help fight cancer and heart disease / by
Gail L. Becker; introduction by Gladys Block. — 1st ed.
        p.   cm.
    ISBN 0-8129-2143-7
    1. Vitamins in human nutrition.   2. Antioxidants.
3. Food—Vitamin content.   I. Title.
QP771.B38   1993
613.2'8—dc20   92-50496

Manufactured in the United States of America
9 8 7 6 5 4 3 2
First Edition
DESIGNED BY ANISTATIA R. MILLER

ACKNOWLEDGMENTS

I would like to thank Annette R. Schottenfeld, M.B.A., R.D., for her assistance in nutrition research and nutritional analyses, and Meryl Hechtman for her contribution to the preparation of this book.

CONTENTS

INTRODUCTION
GLADYS BLOCK, PH.D.

Your mother was right when she told you to eat your fruits and vegetables. What she never told you was why these foods were so good for you. Even now, scientists are discovering more about the foods we eat and how they affect our health.

Epidemiological studies, which examine the relationship between a person's behavior and the risk of various diseases, have found that people with diets rich in fruits and vegetables containing vitamin C, beta carotene, and other carotenoids have significantly lower risk of developing cancer and other chronic illnesses. Vitamin E, found mainly in nuts, seeds, and oils, has also exhibited these protective benefits.

Antioxidants, which include vitamins C and E, beta carotene, and other carotenoids, are essential for any organism that lives in an oxygen environment, which includes almost all living things on earth. Most people do not realize that oxygen, while necessary for human life, is also a highly reactive molecule that can damage our body's cells. Natural body processes also generate reactive molecules that can damage cells, body proteins, and DNA. Modern life has added further sources of oxidative damage, such as cigarette smoking, alcohol, and even to some extent, aerobic exercise. Our bodies have numerous repair processes as protection from these processes. The antioxidants from the foods we eat are extremely important in maintaining this defense against oxidative damage.

Nature has made it easy for us to obtain these nutrients that we need. Vitamins, minerals, fiber, and other nutrients are packaged together in many foods, literally making variety the spice of life. Many of these nutrients are synergistic, meaning that they provide more benefits when in combination with each other than when ingested separately. For example, vitamin E and iron supplies are more available for use by the body in the presence of vitamin C.

Many of the diseases we associate with growing older—heart disease, cancer, cataracts, even the "normal" consequences of aging itself—may be caused by an accumulation of oxidative damage. Studies have found that antioxidants improve the functioning of our disease-fighting immune system. They also prevent some of the changes in arteries that can lead to heart attacks, and even reduce cancer risk. Some studies have found that people whose diets are rich in antioxidants have better mental functioning.

So why do Americans still fall short on obtaining many nutrients? Until recently, most people were relatively unaware of the scientific evidence linking diet and health. People frequently claim to be "too busy" to consume adequate amounts of fruits and vegetables, although these foods are among the easiest to prepare or snack on. Perhaps the major reason we don't consume enough antioxidants is that we aren't sure what they are and how to incorporate them into our diets. This guide was written to help you solve the antioxidant puzzle. It contains information that will help you to recognize antioxidants, make better food choices, and develop healthier lifestyle dietary choices. So read, enjoy, and thank your mom for all that good advice.

—Gladys Block, Ph.D.,
nutritional epidemiologist and professor of
public health nutrition, University of California
at Berkeley; former epidemiologist for the
Division of Cancer Prevention and Control at
the National Cancer Institute

THE
ANTIOXIDANT
POCKET COUNTER

1

PREVENTING DISEASE: THE DIET CONNECTION

Antioxidants. Fiber. Saturated fat. The "Eating Right Pyramid." These aren't things any of us ever thought about ten or fifteen years ago. Back then, we ate bacon and eggs for breakfast, a hamburger and french fries for lunch, and a steak dinner with all the trimmings without a second thought. Today, thanks—or maybe no thanks!—to modern research and public awareness, we're much more knowledgeable about the foods we eat.

We're also much more aware that what we eat can have a tremendous influence on our health. In fact, the evidence is overwhelming that diet plays a significant role in four of the top ten killers in the United States: heart disease, cancer, stroke, and diabetes mellitus.

We all want to live longer—and better. The problem is, it's difficult to put today's headlines into practical use. As a registered dietitian for over twenty years, I've spent a lot of time helping people learn how to use the latest scientific findings to eat more healthfully and make other important life-style changes.

In this guide, I'm going to show you how to make the most current nutritional research work for you. I'm going to focus on what scientists are now learning about how certain vitamins—the antioxidants, which I'll discuss in detail later—and other pivotal nutrients play important roles in contributing to reducing the risk from this country's two biggest killers: heart disease and cancer. And, while there are no magical remedies or guarantees to ward off these diseases, you will learn that by incorporating more antioxidants and fiber into your diet and eating less fat, you can take significant steps toward prevention.

Some experts estimate that a third or more of all cases of heart disease and cancer may be directly related to diet. Leading health authorities, such as the American Cancer Society, the American Heart Association, the National Cancer Institute, and United States Department of Agriculture/Department of Health and Human Services, have issued dietary recommendations based on current scientific information that acknowledge the connection between diet and disease prevention. This guide will help you follow those recommendations and will provide you with tables that show exactly how much of certain key nutrients are present in the foods you eat.

While what we eat has a tremendous influence on our health, diet is only one factor we need to consider. Some of the other life-style changes that the United States Department of Health and Human Services recommends you follow are: do moderate exercise daily, don't smoke, maintain an appropriate weight, protect yourself from job hazards, and get regular medical checkups.

Changing lifelong habits does not occur overnight. I will show you how you can slowly adapt to a more healthful life-style. You may be surprised at how easy it can be. So, read on and learn how to take an important step toward maximizing your health potential by getting more essential nutrients into your diet. This is your chance to really make a difference!

Before we begin, an important word of caution. Never assume that "if some is good, more is better" when you're taking vitamins. Some vitamins can be toxic and have very serious side effects if taken at too-high doses for an extended period of time, particularly if you are pregnant. Share this guide with your doctor so he or she can help you reach your health goals and be sure you're consuming the right amount of nutrients depending on your state of health. I hope this book will help you and your doctor form a happy partnership as you work toward better health.

AN OUNCE OF PREVENTION

Many factors influence your susceptibility to chronic illness, particularly cancer and heart disease: your genetic heritage, age, and gender among them. You can't change those things. But you have the power to adopt a positive life-style, which can help protect you from chronic disease. You have the choice. Don't let yourself become one of the many Americans who are aware of preventive life-style factors, but fail to follow through on them.

For example, while the negative health effects of smoking have been well documented, approximately 25 million men and 22 million women in the United States continue to smoke, placing themselves at greater risk for heart disease and certain types of cancer.

Americans have also been slow to make healthful changes in their diets. We have all heard leading health authorities' recommendations to consume at least five servings of fruit and vegetables per day, yet it is estimated that only 10 percent of us actually do so.

Studies in the last few years have revolutionized our understanding of the role of dietary components, such as antioxidants, dietary fiber, and fat, as they influence health. Let me explain why these nutrients are so important. Let's start by looking at the antioxidants.

ANTIOXIDANTS

What are antioxidants? How do they work? What benefits can they offer? Antioxidants are substances found naturally in your body that react with foreign elements to neutralize their potentially harmful effects. Specifically, antioxidants protect cells from damage caused by *free radicals*, highly reactive chemical substances that are produced during oxidation, the body's normal process of burning fuel for energy. Free radicals are generated in normal body processes and even have some essential functions. For example, they assist germ-killing cells in fighting off certain types of bacteria. However, they are also caused by exposure to hazardous elements such as cigarette smoke and other carcinogens, pollution and environmental toxins, exhaust fumes, radiation, excessive sunlight, and certain medications. The reaction of free radicals with oxygen is what causes butter and vegetable oil to turn rancid, fruit to turn brown, and metal to rust. It can cause the same type of damage in your body. When your body produces too many free radicals, the process leads to a damaging chain reaction in which the free radicals kill or maim the body's cells by attacking their membranes and genetic material, damaging DNA, and altering biochemical compounds. Such damage can eventually contribute to certain neurological disorders and degenerative diseases, including cancer, cystic fibrosis, and cataracts.

Antioxidants help counter the effects of these damages. Although our bodies have their own supply of antioxidants, studies indicate that increasing your intake of certain nutrients may provide added protection against the destructive effect of free radicals. The results of research conducted at major health centers nationwide suggest nutrient levels well above the current U.S. Recommended Daily Allowances (U.S. RDA) that safeguard against nutritional deficiencies.

Vitamins are nutrients required to help our bodies digest, absorb, and utilize food for energy. Minerals are elements that assist in specific chemical reactions to help maintain normal health and body function. Several vitamins and minerals have been cited for their antioxidant benefits, including vitamins C and E and beta carotene, and compounds similar to beta carotene called carotenoids. These antioxidants have been shown to reduce the risk of chronic diseases such as cancer, heart disease, and rheumatoid arthritis, and conditions related to aging, such as cataracts. Both vitamin A, a weak antioxidant, and vitamin E are fat-soluble vitamins, which can't be absorbed by the body unless there is some fat present in the digestive tract. Like fats, fat-soluble vitamins tend to be digested and then stored in the body. Beta carotene is also fat-soluble, but it occurs in a water-soluble form in many vegetables and fruits. A small portion becomes vitamin A in your body; and this production is carefully limited. Beta carotene in most supplements is *not* water-soluble, but fat-soluble. Vitamin C is water-soluble and is not usually stored in the body, which uses the amount of the nutrient it needs and eliminates the rest. Since our bodies can't produce these nutrients, we must obtain them through our diet. Let's briefly review these antioxidants, which work in concert to promote good health.

VITAMIN A
AND BETA CAROTENE

Vitamin A is a fat-soluble vitamin that is necessary for vision, reproduction, growth, and healthy skin, hair, and body tissues. Although vitamin A is not a very active antioxidant, it helps your body resist infection and has been shown to reduce the incidence of cancer. Preformed or actual vitamin A, also known as retinol, can be used by the body in its given form and is found in animal food (such as meat, egg, and dairy) products. Some foods, such as butter and margarine, are fortified with vitamin A. Other good sources of vitamin A include liver, eggs, cheese, and fish oils. All of these sources, however, are generally high in fat and/or cholesterol. Vitamin A can also be obtained from foods containing beta carotene, a related nutrient and antioxidant, which I discuss below.

How much vitamin A do you require? We have all

heard the terms RDA (Recommended Dietary Allowances) and U.S. RDA (U.S. Recommended Daily Allowances), but you may not be sure of the exact difference between these two nutrient standards set by the government. The RDAs are average daily recommended intakes of nutrients (calories and certain vitamins and minerals), for specific age groups that are intended to provide a margin of safety to meet all healthy individuals' nutrient needs in the United States. On the other hand, the U.S. RDA is a single recommended nutrient value used for food labeling purposes and usually represents the highest number for each nutrient recommended in the RDA table.

The U.S. RDA for vitamin A is 5,000 I.U. (International Units) per day. Some experts suggest that you aim for more than this level for added protection, especially if you smoke cigarettes. You should remember, though, that vitamin A, like all fat-soluble vitamins, can be stored by the body and excessive intake can be toxic, causing such symptoms as dry skin, fatigue, blurred vision, liver damage, and harm to the fetus if you are pregnant. Your normal daily intake should not exceed 25,000 I.U. over an extended period of time without the supervision of your doctor.

To meet your daily requirement for vitamin A, you could select foods such as the following: 1 cup lowfat or nonfat milk (500 I.U.), 1 cup lowfat or nonfat vanilla yogurt (862 I.U.), 1 cup minestrone soup (1,113 I.U.), 3 medium fresh apricots (1,109 I.U.), and 1 slice pumpkin bread (3,418 I.U.). Much of the vitamin A we obtain in our diets is obtained from foods high in beta carotene, which is converted into vitamin A in the body. It is important, though, to select occasionally some foods that are good sources of vitamin A (e.g., nonfat milk products, eggs, liver) for the nutrients they contain, which may not be present in foods high in beta carotene (e.g., certain fruits and vegetables).

Beta carotene is a related antioxidant that is partially converted into vitamin A in the body. It is one of the over 400 carotenoid pigments, all with antioxidant properties, that give color to yellow-orange fruits and vegetables such as cantaloupe and carrots and are also present in green leafy vegetables such as spinach. Beta carotene's preventive benefits are most strongly related to its naturally occurring form, as opposed to when it is converted to vitamin A.

Beta carotene has shown protective effects against certain forms of cancer, including lung, stomach, colon, prostate, and cervical cancer. One study at the University of Texas followed male smokers over a nineteen-year period and found that those who ate the fewest foods containing beta carotene were eight times more likely to develop lung cancer than those whose diets were high in beta carotene. Another significant study, of 2,974 male subjects conducted in Basel, Switzerland, and ongoing since 1959, found an increased overall cancer risk when plasma (blood) carotene and retinol levels were low.

Diets high in beta carotene have also been found to protect against cataracts, enhance the immune system, treat some light-sensitive skin disorders, and reduce the risk of heart disease. The Physicians' Health Study, a ten-year study of over 22,000 male physicians by Harvard Medical School, found that the subjects who had previous histories of heart disease benefited from beta carotene supplements of 50 milligrams every other day. The 333 people in this group experienced half as many heart attacks, strokes, and deaths as those on placebo pills. In a separate ongoing study of over 87,000 female nurses, participants whose diets were highest in beta carotene had a 22 percent lower risk of heart attack and 40 percent lower risk of stroke than women with diets low in beta carotene.

Many carotenoids, compounds similar to beta carotene, are abundant in fruits and vegetables. These carotenoids, such as lutein and lycopene, are also effective antioxidants and have been shown in epidemiologic studies to reduce cancer risk. Since they don't come in a pill, you need to eat fruits and vegetables to obtain them.

How much beta carotene is right for you? Although there is no Recommended Dietary Allowance (RDA) for beta carotene, diets suggested by the U.S. Department of Agriculture and the National Cancer Institute would provide about 5–6 milligrams of beta carotene per day. This amounts to one or two servings of beta carotene–rich food every day. If you are a smoker, use oral contraceptives, or are frequently outdoors (where you're exposed to environmental toxins and the ultraviolet rays of the sun), your need for beta carotene will be higher than that of individuals not exposed to these factors.

Unlike preformed vitamin A, a high intake of beta carotene does not lead to toxic side effects. And, since beta carotene can be partially converted to vitamin A in the body, eating foods high in beta carotene is a safe way to get extra vitamin A. However, if you consume large amounts of beta carotene over a period of time, your skin may turn an orange-yellow color. This effect is harmless and will disappear if you decrease your intake of the antioxidant. Most people currently consume an average of only 1.5 milligrams of beta carotene daily. Using your nutrition smarts you will see how easy it is to meet your

11

daily beta carotene needs. For example, by selecting ½ cup dried apricots (3 milligrams) at breakfast, ½ cup cooked carrots at lunch (6 milligrams), 1 cup vegetable juice cocktail (2 milligrams) at dinner, and ½ medium cantaloupe (8 milligrams) for a snack, you have more then met your beta carotene needs (total = 19 milligrams). You should make a concerted effort to fill the "beta carotene gap" and select good sources of beta carotene, such as the ones listed below.

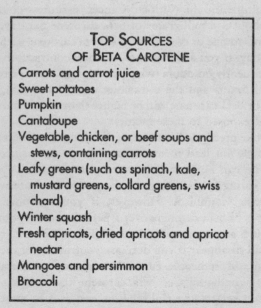

TOP SOURCES
OF BETA CAROTENE

Carrots and carrot juice

Sweet potatoes

Pumpkin

Cantaloupe

Vegetable, chicken, or beef soups and
stews, containing carrots

Leafy greens (such as spinach, kale,
mustard greens, collard greens, swiss
chard)

Winter squash

Fresh apricots, dried apricots and apricot
nectar

Mangoes and persimmon

Broccoli

VITAMIN C

Vitamin C, a familiar nutrient, is another antioxidant. Also known as ascorbic acid, vitamin C has many important functions, including enhancing iron absorption, producing collagen (part of the skin that maintains its integrity), assisting in wound healing, and stimulating the immune system.

Vitamin C may also play a role in preventing heart disease by lowering blood pressure, raising levels of "good" cholesterol—high-density lipoproteins, or HDLs —and preventing the oxidation of "bad" cholesterol— low-density lipoproteins, or LDLs, which can lead to plaque buildup in the arteries. Investigators with the National Institute on Aging found in a study involving more than 550 men and 300 women that those with the highest vitamin C blood values also had higher levels of HDLs. Two other recent studies conducted by researchers at the U.S. Department of Agriculture's Nutrition Research Center on Aging indicated that of the 600 elderly subjects, those with higher levels of vitamin C consistently had lower blood pressure. And, researchers from the University of California at Los Angeles found that vitamin C significantly lowered total mortality and heart-disease mortality in a follow-up study of over eleven thousand Americans from the First National Health and Nutrition Examination Survey (known as NHANES I).

A recent analysis of over ninety scientific studies reinforced strong evidence that vitamin C may also help prevent certain forms of cancer, including oral, stomach, esophageal, pancreatic, lung, and rectal cancers. One study in Finland of 4,538 men aged 20 to 69 years conducted over a twenty-year period found that among the subjects who were nonsmokers, there was a higher incidence of lung cancer among those with low intakes of beta carotene, vitamin C, and vitamin E. Vitamin C also appears to prevent the formation of cataracts later in life by protecting the cornea from ultraviolet light.

How much vitamin C do you need? Since vitamin C is a water-soluble vitamin, your body will use what it needs and eliminate the rest. Since you can't store this vitamin in your body, you need to consume some vitamin C–rich foods every day. It has not been found to be toxic at high levels, but can produce stomachaches and diarrhea at extremely high levels such as 10,000 milligrams. The U.S. RDA for vitamin C is 60 milligrams per day. Although this level is adequate to prevent vitamin C deficiency (scurvy), scientists don't know the optimum levels for disease prevention. If you smoke cigarettes, take oral contraceptive pills, or lead a stressful life, your vitamin C requirement may be higher. Studies have shown that vitamin C levels in the blood of smokers are 20–40 percent lower than those of nonsmokers. If you consume at least five servings of vitamin C–rich fruits and vegetables daily, you will receive about 200 milligrams of the vitamin. Since researchers recommend even higher levels for preventive benefits, try selecting good sources of vitamin C each day. Though citrus fruits are excellent sources of vitamin C, the chart below will show you that there are many other ways to get your "C." As an added bonus, several of these foods are also good sources of beta carotene and other carotenoids.

TOP SOURCES
OF VITAMIN C

Melons (especially cantaloupe)
Citrus fruits and juices (such as oranges
    and grapefruits)
Red and green peppers
Leafy greens (such as mustard greens,
    turnip greens, kale and collards)
Strawberries
Papaya, kiwi, and mangoes
Cruciferous vegetables (broccoli,
    cauliflower, brussels sprouts, kohlrabi,
    cabbage)
Fortified cereals
Tomatoes and tomato juice
Sweet potatoes, with skin
Blackberries and raspberries

VITAMIN E

The last antioxidant I will discuss is vitamin E, also referred to as tocopherol. Like beta carotene and vitamin C, vitamin E is believed to reduce the risk of heart disease and degenerative disorders such as cataracts, cancer, and immune-function disorders. In one ongoing study of over 87,000 female nurses, the Nurses' Health Study, subjects with the highest vitamin E intake, 100 milligrams or more daily, experienced a 36 percent reduction in the risk of heart attack and a 23 percent reduction in risk of stroke.

Other studies have shown vitamin E's benefits in preventing certain types of cancer, including cancer of the stomach, bladder, breast, colon, rectum, and lung. One large study, the Finnish Mobile Clinic Health Survey, followed 36,265 individuals from twenty-five population groups in different parts of Finland for twelve years. The subjects with low serum vitamin E levels had about one and a half times the risk of developing cancer compared with those who had higher serum vitamin E levels.

How much vitamin E should you consume every day? The U.S. RDA for vitamin E is 30 I.U. (or 20 milligrams) daily. Health professionals recommend greater amounts of 45 I.U. (or 30 milligrams) daily, and research studies have used even higher levels, including 800 I.U. for three years without toxic side effects. If you smoke or are exposed to a lot of pollutants, you may need more vitamin E than suggested by the U.S. RDA.

It is recommended for good health that we decrease the total fat in our diets and select more polyunsaturated fats (PUFA) and monounsaturated fats. Both of these fat types are healthier than the saturated type of fat and I will discuss them later on. Ironically, vegetable oils that are high in PUFA decrease vitamin E availability, but these oils are good sources of vitamin E so the effect is somewhat balanced out with moderate intake. Other factors that can increase your need for this antioxidant are pollution and smoking. Food selections that could easily fit into your diet and meet your daily vitamin E requirement include, for an example of 27 milligrams of vitamin E: ¼ cup wheat germ (5 milligrams), 1 medium mango (2 milligrams), ¼ cup hazelnuts (8 milligrams), 3 ounces cooked shrimp (2 milligrams), ½ cup cooked spinach (2 milligrams), and 1 tablespoon sunflower oil (8 milligrams). Try to select foods from the following chart to obtain good sources of vitamin E in your daily diet. The chart on pp. 18–19 summarizes the recommended amounts of antioxidant vitamins and factors that can affect your need for them. Although the U.S. RDAs are intended for adults and children over 4 years of age, the RDA for children are usually lower for most vitamins. Ask your pediatrician about your child's vitamin needs. Remember: amounts that are safe for adults could be toxic for children. While there is no U.S. RDA for beta carotene, the U.S. Department of Agriculture and the National Cancer Institute recommend a diet that provides approximately 5–6 milligrams of beta carotene per day.

TOP SOURCES OF VITAMIN E

Seeds
Nuts and peanut butter
Vegetable oils
Mayonnaise
Wheat germ
Leafy greens (such as fresh spinach, kale,
    and collard greens)
Fish and shellfish
Avocados
Mangoes
Whole grain products
Fortified cereals

Nutrient	Type	U.S. RDA	Conservative Recommendations to Help Prevent Cancer	Factors That Can Increase Nutrient Requirements	Sample Foods to Meet Requirements
Vitamin A	Fat-soluble vitamin	5,000 I.U.	12,500 I.U.	smoking	1 cup low-fat or nonfat milk (500 I.U.) 1 cup low-fat or nonfat vanilla yogurt (311 I.U.) 1 cup vegetable stew (15,717 I.U.)
Beta Carotene and Other Carotenoids	Vitamin A precursor	none	5–6 mg	smoking oral contraceptives U.V. light	½ cup dried apricots (3 mg) ½ cup red pepper (2 mg) ½ cup cooked spinach (4 mg) ½ medium cantaloupe (8 mg)

18

Vitamin C	Water-soluble vitamin	60 mg	1,000 mg	smoking environmental and emotional stress oral contraceptives aerobic exercise alcohol	1 cup mandarin orange sections (25 mg) 1 medium grapefruit (100 mg) ½ cup cooked broccoli (37 mg) 1 cup tomato soup (133 mg)
Vitamin E	Fat-soluble vitamin	30 I.U.* (20 mg)	300–800 I.U. (133–533 mg)	high intake of polyunsaturated fats pollution smoking aerobic exercise	¼ cup wheat germ (5 mg) 1 tbs. sunflower oil (8 mg) ¼ cup almonds (6 mg) 3 ounces cooked shrimp (2 mg)

*30 I.U. vitamin E = 20 mg vitamin E

SOURCE: Adapted from R. R. Watson and T. K. Leonard, "Selenium and Vitamins A, E, and C: Nutrients with Cancer Prevention Properties," *Journal of the American Dietetic Association*, Vol. 86, no. 4, 1986.

Remember "vitamins A, C, and E and beta carotene" to keep you healthy!

DO YOU NEED TO TAKE A VITAMIN SUPPLEMENT?

Now that you understand how important antioxidants are, wouldn't it be easiest simply to take a vitamin pill every day to be sure you get the amounts you need? Remember, a vitamin supplement may be appropriate "insurance," but it should never be used to replace healthful foods. And don't fall into the trap of thinking that more is better. Taken at too high dosages, vitamins can have harmful side effects.

The best way to ensure you are fulfilling your nutrition requirements is to eat a varied diet emphasizing foods considered to be significant sources of vitamins A, C, E and beta carotene, among other nutrients. However, it should be noted that most of the foods high in vitamin E are also high in fat. You should therefore strongly consider taking a vitamin E supplement. A varied diet is the best way to ensure adequate intake of nutrients that work in concert to enhance each other's effectiveness. For example, adding a few slices of vitamin C–rich tomato to a hamburger increases the absorption of iron from the meat. A varied diet also provides you with the calories, roughage (fiber), minerals, and sense of satiety—not to mention pleasure—that a vitamin supplement can't provide.

However, although eating a well-balanced diet provides the foundation for maximizing the potential health benefits these nutrients offer, many people today don't do it. A hectic life-style, vacations, business lunches—all these and more can sabotage the most healthful of intentions. If this sounds like your life, you may want to take vitamin and mineral supplements as extra insurance to fill in the "nutritional gaps." You should also talk to your doctor about taking vitamin supplements if you have special dietary needs, are pregnant, nursing, have food allergies, or cannot tolerate certain foods (e.g., lactose intolerance), or are older, or if you're a smoker, or are restricting calories to control your weight.

Most scientific studies investigating nutrients to prevent disease use dosage levels above the U.S. RDA. I suggest you consult with a health professional who can help you assess your nutritional needs and use this handy guide to evaluate if your diet provides you with these vital nutrients. Then consider dietary supplements to fill in the "nutritional gaps."

THE FACTS ON FIBER AND FAT

If your goal is to help prevent illness, adding antioxidants alone to your diet may not be enough. You should know that there are many other components of your diet that can impact your health. Three of these important components are dietary fiber, cholesterol, and fat.

Dietary Fiber

A wealth of scientific evidence, including a recent study at Harvard University's School of Public Health, also supports the benefits of consuming foods rich in dietary fiber to reduce the risk of some types of cancer, particularly cancer of the colon and rectum.

Dietary fiber is found in plant cells and is nondigestible. There are two forms of fiber—soluble and insoluble—that offer different health benefits. Soluble fiber dissolves in water and can be effective for lowering blood cholesterol. Sources include dried beans, peas, oats, barley fruits, vegetables, and supplements. Insoluble fiber does not dissolve in water and helps to increase bulk and aid in regularity. This type of fiber has also been linked to lowering the risk of colon and rectum cancer. Some health authorities believe this is because fiber speeds up the time it takes food to pass through the intestines, shortening the amount of time cancer-causing agents from foods remain in the body. Insoluble fiber can be found in whole grains and brans of wheat, rye, and rice, vegetables, and fruits with edible seeds (e.g., strawberries).

How much dietary fiber should you eat? The experts recommend increasing both types of fiber in your diet so that you obtain an average total dietary fiber intake of 20–35 grams per day (most Americans consume only about 10–12 grams per day). When increasing your dietary fiber intake, do so gradually and make sure to drink plenty of fluids to help in digestion and elimination of body wastes. Add more fiber to your diet by selecting whole-grain breads, cereals, and pastas in place of white breads and highly processed cereals and pastas, choosing brown rice in place of white rice, and fresh or dried fruits, raw vegetables, or air-popped popcorn as snacks in place of chips, cookies, and candy. The following chart lists foods high in dietary fiber that you can incorporate into your meals to achieve the recommended goal of 20–35 grams of dietary fiber per day. For example, by selecting 1 medium grapefruit (4 grams) and ¼ cup wheat germ (4 grams) as part of your breakfast, 1 medium apple with skin (3 grams) and 2 slices rye bread (4 grams) at lunch, ½ cup lima beans (7 grams) and ½ cup broccoli (3 grams) at dinner and ¼ cup almonds (3 grams) as a snack, you have more then met your dietary fiber requirements for the day (total = 28 grams).

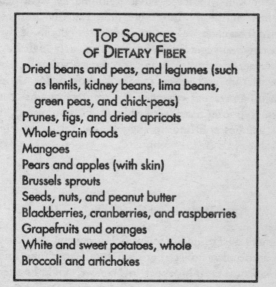

TOP SOURCES OF DIETARY FIBER

Dried beans and peas, and legumes (such as lentils, kidney beans, lima beans, green peas, and chick-peas)

Prunes, figs, and dried apricots

Whole-grain foods

Mangoes

Pears and apples (with skin)

Brussels sprouts

Seeds, nuts, and peanut butter

Blackberries, cranberries, and raspberries

Grapefruits and oranges

White and sweet potatoes, whole

Broccoli and artichokes

Cruciferous Vegetables

Cruciferous vegetables, members of the cabbage family, are good sources of dietary fiber and vitamins, including antioxidants such as vitamin C and beta carotene, and are low in calories. Examples include broccoli, brussels sprouts, cabbage, cauliflower, kale, kohlrabi, mustard greens, and Swiss chard. Studies have suggested that cruciferous vegetables play a role in reducing the risk of colon and certain other cancers, but for more than fifteen years it was not known why. More recently, studies, conducted by researchers at John Hopkins University School of Medicine, have preliminarily identified the chemical that may be responsible for this anti-cancer benefit. The chemical, known as sulforaphane, is present in cruciferous vegetables and is particularly high in broccoli. Other vegetables found to contain sulforaphane include carrots and green onions. Sulforaphane seems to work by activating enzymes that protect against cancer. Although more research needs to be completed, these initial studies continue to suggest that eating cruciferous vegetables is a healthy choice.

Cholesterol and Fats

There is significant scientific agreement that a strong association exists between total fat intake and the risk of certain types of cancer, including colon, breast, and prostate cancer. A study conducted at the Harvard University School of Public Health found that the risk of colon cancer for women who ate the most animal fat was almost double compared to that of women who ate the least.

A high-fat diet has also been found to contribute to the

risk of strokes and heart disease, because fat increases body weight and saturated fat and cholesterol (a fatlike substance) contribute to the buildup of fat in the body's arteries.

What is the maximum amount of cholesterol and fat you can eat each day? Limit your dietary cholesterol to 300 milligrams or less per day. Cholesterol is found in animal food products only; grains, fruits, and vegetables do not contain cholesterol unless it is added to them. Foods that are highest in cholesterol, and should be limited to about three servings per week, include: organ meats, whole-milk dairy products, and egg yolks. Currently, the average American's diet contains about 36–37 percent of calories from total fat. Health professionals recommend that you consume 30 percent or less of your daily calories from total fat, 10 percent or less from saturated fat, and eat a high-fiber diet.

As a rule of thumb, saturated fats are usually those that are solid at room temperature (e.g., lard) and have been shown to contribute to fatty buildup in the arteries. Poly-unsaturated and monounsaturated fats are usually liquid at room temperature and don't have the same negative health effects as saturated fats. Remember, the more solid a fat is, the more saturated it usually is. When reading food labels that provide the fat content, select only those that have at least a 2:1 ratio of polyunsaturated to saturated fat grams (twice as much polyunsaturated fat). Use the following as a quick reference in determining whether a food product contains too much fat to fit into your daily fat allowance.

The first step in determining your appropriate dietary fat limit is to calculate your daily calorie needs. Remember, dietary fat has 9 calories per gram as opposed to 4 calories per gram for carbohydrate and protein. Calorie requirements are based on body size, height, age, sex, and activity level. To determine your personal daily calorie requirement to achieve or maintain ideal weight, use the following guidelines:

1. Calculate your *basal calorie requirement* (the energy used at rest) by multiplying your personal weight goal or ideal weight (see chart p. 34) by one of the following factors:

Age	Women	Men
under 45	10	11
over 45	9	10

2. Adjust calorie requirements for age by subtracting 10 calories for each year over 25 from your basal energy requirement (from 1).
3. Add calories for physical activity by multiplying the above figure (from 2) by one of the following:

   * sedentary (office work): 1.3
   * moderately sedentary
     (occasional exercise): 1.4
   * moderately active
     (regular exercise): 1.5
   * extremely active
     (training program): 2

   For example, a woman who is 35 years of age, of a small frame, 5 feet 4 inches tall, and moderately sedentary would calculate her caloric requirements as follows:

1. 125 pounds (goal weight) × 10 calories/pound
                                = 1,250 calories
2. 35 years − 25 years   = 10 years
      10 years × 10 calories/year   = 100 calories
      1,250 calories − 100 calories = 1,150 calories
3. 1,150 calories × 1.4   = 1,610 calories

DAILY CALORIES	TOTAL DIETARY FAT LIMIT	ALLOWANCE OF SATURATED FAT
1,500	50 grams/day	17 grams/day
2,000	67 grams/day	22 grams/day
2,500	83 grams/day	28 grams/day

To obtain your Total Dietary Fat Limit, you multiply your total daily calories by 30 percent (.30) and divide this number by 9 calories per gram of fat. For example, if you eat 1,500 calories per day: 1,500 calories × 30 percent of calories from total fat ÷ 9 calories per gram of fat = 50 grams of total fat allowed per day.

To obtain your Allowance of Saturated Fat, you multiply your total daily calories by 10 percent (.10) and divide this number by 9 calories per gram of fat. For example, if you eat 1,500 calories per day: 1,500 calories × 10 percent of calories from saturated fat ÷ 9 calories per gram of fat = 17 grams of saturated fat allowed per day.

Get into the habit of reading food labels to determine the amount of dietary fiber, total fat, and saturated fat in the foods you eat—the next section will show you how. You can also use the handy food tables in this counter to help you make healthier food choices.

2

SELECTING
AND
PREPARING FOODS

REDUCING NUTRIENT LOSS

A great deal happens to food from the time it leaves the farm until it reaches our tables. Selecting foods that will give you the best nutrient value means using your good health smarts. Whole or fresh foods that have been minimally processed are richest in vitamins, minerals, and dietary fiber. In selecting fresh fruits and vegetables, remember to choose those that are free of decay or discoloration; crisp, not wilted or shriveled; free from bruises and blemishes; firm; and plump. This will help to ensure that minimal nutrient damage has occurred. Frozen fruits and vegetables are also good choices, as freezing helps to protect nutrients from being destroyed. Highly processed or canned fruits and vegetables will experience the most nutrient loss because they are exposed to a heating process that can destroy important vitamins. Although canned items are convenient and can be used occasionally, fresh or frozen varieties offer better nutritional value. Dried fruits are also good alternatives, since they are more concentrated and offer high nutrient content. Count how many handfuls you are taking, though, since dried fruits are high in calories.

The most healthful foods can lose their nutritional value before they ever reach your plate because certain vitamins and minerals can be lost or destroyed during cooking. To reduce the nutrient loss of your foods, follow these suggested cooking tips:

- Use acids such as lemon juice, other citrus juices, or vinegar to slow enzyme activity in fruits and vegetables. Enzyme activity (browning) occurs when foods are exposed to oxygen in the air (oxidation) and leads to the destruction of beta carotene, vitamin C, E, and other vitamins.

- If a recipe recommends cutting up foods, leave the pieces as big as possible and don't chop or slice too far in advance of cooking or serving, so as to minimize exposing the surface areas to oxygen and nutrient destruction.

- Refrigerate or freeze foods to slow destructive enzyme activity.

- Do not add baking soda to green vegetables during cooking, since it tends to destroy B vitamins and vitamin C by creating an alkaline medium.

- Use the least amount of water in cooking, so that water-soluble vitamins (B vitamins and vitamin C) and minerals in your foods don't leach out into the cooking water. Steam, stir-fry, or use a microwave or waterless or pressure-cooking methods when cooking vegetables.

• The longer foods are stored or cooked, the more vitamins they generally lose. To shorten cooking times:
  —Cook vegetables only to crisp—not mushy.
  —Cover the pan to keep heat in so you won't have to cook foods so long.
  —Start cooking your foods on a hot pan or hot cooking element or in already rapidly boiling water.

SELECTED COOKING METHODS

Research has shown that cooking methods such as barbecuing, grilling, or smoking can produce carcinogens, cancer-causing substances. Therefore, it is wise to use cooking methods such as roasting or baking that prevent the creation of harmful substances, because foods cook more slowly at lower temperatures. If like most people you enjoy the taste of barbecued or grilled foods, try wrapping food in foil before barbecuing or putting it in a pan so that it does not come into direct contact with the smoke or flames. You might also microwave meat for a few minutes before barbecuing to cut down on cooking time. Opposite is a chart outlining which cooking methods to use more frequently and less frequently.

Try to limit the total amount of fat in the foods you select and prepare. Not all fat is visible, but when it is, trim off all of it before cooking. Remember, even fats that are better for you should not be used in excessive amounts. Try substituting these healthier choices for certain popular foods.

COOKING METHODS TO USE MORE FREQUENTLY
- Baking
- Boiling
- Microwave cooking
- Oven broiling
- Poaching
- Roasting
- Steaming
- Stewing

COOKING METHODS TO USE LESS FREQUENTLY
- Barbecuing
- Charcoal broiling
- Frying
- Grilling
- Smoking

LOW-FAT SUBSTITUTIONS FOR FOOD PREPARATION

INSTEAD OF:	SELECT:
Cheese, whole-milk varieties	Cheese, low-fat or nonfat varieties
Cream	Condensed, nonfat (skim) milk
Eggs, 1 whole	Eggs, 2 whites
Ice cream	Nonfat frozen yogurt
Milk, whole or 2%	Milk, nonfat (skim) or 1%
Oil (in baked goods)	Pureed fruit (such as pureed apricots or applesauce)
Sour cream	Nonfat yogurt, plain

31

3
EXPERT ADVICE

Take it from the experts: Selecting a healthful diet is a vital component of a preventive life-style. Leading health authorities, such as the U.S. Department of Agriculture/Department of Health and Human Services, the American Cancer Society, the American Heart Association, and the National Cancer Institute, have each suggested dietary guidelines for healthy individuals. While each organization's specific guidelines differ, they all recognize that people have different nutrient requirement levels and that a healthful diet consists of the same basic ingredients.

To boil down the overall message from these experts, here is a summary of the *Dietary Guidelines for Americans* suggested by the U.S. Department of Agriculture/Department of Health and Human Services, plus additional recommendations by other health authorities:

- *Eat a variety of foods.* No one food alone can meet all of your nutrient needs. Choose a variety of foods from the different food groups (see p. 38).

- *Maintain a healthy weight.* Obesity (weight of 20 percent or more above your suggested weight) is a risk factor linked with high blood pressure, heart disease, stroke, the most common form of diabetes, certain cancers, and other illnesses. Determine a healthy weight for yourself by using the chart on p. 34. Setting realistic weight loss or maintenance goals, eating a healthful diet, and exercising are steps you can take that will gradually lead you toward maintaining a healthy weight that is right for you.

* *Choose a diet low in fat, saturated fat, and cholesterol.* A diet low in total fat (30 percent or less of your total daily calories from fat) may lower your risk for certain cancers. The American Heart Association also suggests that a lower intake of saturated fat (10 percent or less of your total daily calories) and cholesterol (300 milligrams per day or less) may reduce the risk of heart disease. Instead of using saturated fats, try selecting polyunsaturated and monounsaturated fats to obtain the valuable nutrients they contain.

* *Choose a diet with plenty of vegetables, fruits, and grain products (complex carbohydrates).* Replace the high fats in your diet with complex carbohydrates. Contrary to popular belief, complex carbohydrates are not high in calories or fat, unless they are added to them. These foods offer different types of dietary fiber and various vitamins and minerals. The American Cancer Society recommends that you select a variety of fruits and vegetables every day that are good sources of beta caro-

Suggested Weight for Adults

Height[1]	Weight in Pounds[2,3]	
	19 to 34 Years	35 Years and Over
5'0"	97–128	108–138
5'1"	101–132	111–143
5'2"	104–137	115–148
5'3"	107–141	119–152
5'4"	111–146	122–157
5'5"	114–150	126–162
5'6"	118–155	130–167
5'7"	121–160	134–172
5'8"	125–164	138–178
5'9"	129–169	142–183
5'10"	132–174	146–188
5'11"	136–179	151–194
6'0"	140–184	155–199
6'1"	144–189	159–205
6'2"	148–195	164–210
6'3"	152–200	168–216
6'4"	156–205	173–222
6'5"	160–211	177–228
6'6"	164–216	182–234

1. Without shoes.
2. Without clothes.
3. The higher weight in the ranges generally apply to men, who tend to have more muscle and bone; the lower weights more often apply to women, who have less muscle and bone.

Source: *Nutrition and Your Health: Dietary Guidelines for Americans.* U.S. Department of Agriculture and U.S. Department of Health and Human Services, Home and Garden Bulletin no. 232, 3rd ed., 1990.

Fat type	Primary Sources
Saturated	• Meats • Butter, cream, whole-milk dairy products • Lard, chicken fat • Palm oil • Coconut oil • Cocoa butter
Polyunsaturated	• Safflower oil • Sunflower oil • Corn oil • Soybean oil • Cottonseed oil • Margarines, soft (liquid vegetable oil as first ingredient) • Walnuts • Sunflower seeds, pumpkin seeds, sesame seeds
Monounsaturated	• Canola oil • Olive oil • Peanut oil • Avocado • Almonds, cashews, peanuts, pecans, pistachio nuts
Cholesterol	• Red meats • Organ meats (e.g., liver, kidney) • Egg yolks • Whole-milk dairy products

tene and vitamin C, plus cruciferous (cabbage family) vegetables. These complex carbohydrates have been associated with a lowered incidence of cancer and heart disease. Select at least five fruit and vegetable servings and at least six starch servings per day. Remember, don't spoil a good thing by adding large amounts of fat to your healthy carbohydrates. A freshly steamed dish of broccoli doesn't need a pat of butter to taste delicious.

- *Use sugars only in moderation.* Foods high in sugar (simple carbohydrates) are also high in calories and provide little nutritional value. Try to select foods with little added sugar and avoid cereals with more than 5 grams of sugar per serving. Save sugar treats (e.g., jelly beans) for an occasional snack.

- *Use salt and sodium only in moderation.* Although sodium is an essential mineral in the body, too much sodium and salt (sodium chloride) have been linked to an increased risk of hypertension in some individuals. The National Research Council of the National Academy of Sciences (the group responsible for setting the Recommended Dietary Allowances, or RDAs) suggests a "safe and adequate" range of about 1,100 to 3,300 milligrams (1.1–3.3 grams) of sodium per day for adults. The American Heart Association recommends no more than 3,000 milligrams (3 grams) of sodium per day. Remember, one teaspoon of salt contains about 2,000 milligrams of sodium. Most processed and convenience foods are high in sodium and should be eaten in limited amounts. Surprisingly, large amounts of sodium are also found in items such as baking soda and powder, dark-colored sodas, cheeses, milk, and antacids, and not so surprisingly in seafood, snack foods, commercial soups, condiments such as catsup and soy sauce, and canned meats and vegetables. The American Cancer Society also recommends limiting consumption of salt-cured, smoked, and nitrite-cured foods, which have been linked to certain types of cancer, such as cancer of the stomach and esophagus. Try choosing more fresh fruits and vegetables, using herbs and spices other than salt on foods and in cooking, and making foods from scratch or looking for low-salt versions of favorite foods.

- *Drink alcoholic beverages in moderation, if you drink at all.* Alcohol is high in calories (7 calories per gram versus 4 calories per gram of protein and carbohydrate) and contains little nutritional value. It has also been linked to increased risk of many cancers, cirrhosis of the liver, and many preventable causes of death each year.

Below is a summary chart of the general dietary recommendations from leading health authorities. These recommendations present the range of the dietary guidelines put out by the following leading health authorities: the American Cancer Society, the American Heart Association, the National Cancer Institute, and the U.S. Department of

Agriculture/Department of Health and Human Services. By modifying your diet to adopt these recommendations, you'll be getting all the antioxidants and fiber you need, and less of the fat you probably already get too much of.

DIETARY RECOMMENDATIONS FROM LEADING HEALTH AUTHORITIES		
FOOD GROUP	TOTAL DAILY SERVINGS	SUGGESTED SERVING SIZE
Fruits and vegetables	5 or more (making sure to select deep-yellow/orange fruits and vegetables and green leafy vegetables daily)	· 1 medium whole fruit (such as an apple or orange) · ½ grapefruit · ¾ cup of juice · ½ cup cooked or canned fruit · 1 cup raw leafy vegetables · ½ cup cooked vegetables
Milk products (low-fat or nonfat)	2 or more (3 or more for teens and pregnant or breastfeeding women)	· 1 cup milk or yogurt · 1½ ounces natural cheese · 2 ounces processed cheese

DIETARY RECOMMENDATIONS FROM LEADING HEALTH AUTHORITIES

FOOD GROUP	TOTAL DAILY SERVINGS	SUGGESTED SERVING SIZE
Whole-grain/ enriched breads, cereals, pasta and starchy vegetables	6 or more	· 1 slice bread · ½ bun or roll or bagel · ½ cup cooked cereal, pasta, or rice · 1 ounce dry cereal
Lean meat, fish and poultry, dry beans and peas, eggs, nuts and seeds	2 to 3 servings (limit egg yolks to 2 to 3 yolks or less per week)	· 6 ounces total per day of cooked lean meat, fish, or poultry · Nonmeat substitutions (each equal to 1 ounce of meat, fish, or poultry): —1 whole egg or 2 egg whites —½ cup cooked beans —2 Tbs. peanut butter
Fats and oils	limit depending on calorie needs	· 1 tsp. oil, margarine, or butter · 1 Tbs. mayonnaise or salad dressing

4

How to Use This Guide

Maintaining a diet that will help you fight the effects of aging and chronic disease is easy once you learn the basics for making wise food choices. With this in mind, I designed the handy nutrient guide to help you select foods considered good sources of beta carotene and other carotenoids, vitamins A, C and E, and dietary fiber. The guide also provides the total fat, saturated fat, and calorie content of more than four hundred food items.

But knowing the right foods to eat is only the beginning. Let's now look at some practical tips for reading food labels, creating a shopping list, and developing a healthful meal plan that fits into your life-style.

THE LOWDOWN ON FOOD LABELS

Familiarizing yourself with what is on food labels is key to maintaining a healthful diet. Among the things to look for are nutrient values per serving,

fat, sodium, and dietary fiber content. Many food product labels do not include breakdowns of less frequently
specified nutrients such as beta carotene. The food tables
included in this guide will help you round out the nutritional profiles of many foods by specifying the amount of
each antioxidant and more. In the meantime, use the
guidelines on p. 42 to evaluate the overall goodness of
food products.

Learning the language of labels is easy once you know
what to look for. Here are some tips:

- *Serving size and number of servings in the package.*
  When comparing products, make sure to use the
  same serving amount; these may vary from one
  product to another. You also need to determine if
  the manufacturer's idea of a serving is realistic.
  You may need to multiply the information by one
  and a half, two, or even three, to arrive at the
  serving you actually eat. Recommended serving
  sizes are provided in the table on pp. 38–39.

- *Percentage of calories from total fat and saturated
  fat.* Use this handy formula to determine how
  much fat a product contains: Multiply the number
  of fat grams per serving stated on the label by 9 (the
  number of calories per gram of fat). Divide this
  number of total fat calories by the number of total
  calories per serving. Multiply your answer by 100.
  (For example, 2 grams fat × 9 calories per gram of
  fat = 18 calories from fat per slice ÷ 100 calories
  per slice = .18 × 100 = 18% calories from fat.)
  Then do the same thing using the number of satu-

NUTRIENT	RECOMMENDED AMOUNT
Beta carotene	At least 5 to 6 milligrams per day
Vitamin A	At least 5,000 I.U.* per day (12,500 I.U. per day preventive recommendation)
Vitamin C	At least 60 mg* per day (1,000 mg per day preventive recommendation)
Vitamin E	At least 30 I.U. (20 mg)* per day (300 to 800 I.U. [133–533 mg] per day preventive recommendation)
Dietary Fiber	Approximately 20–35 grams per day
Total Fat	Depends on calorie needs (see pages 26–27)
Saturated Fat	Depends on calorie needs (see pages 26–27)
Cholesterol	Less than 300 mg per day
Sodium	Less than 3,000 mg per day

*The value represents the U.S. RDA for that nutrient.

rated-fat grams; if saturated-fat grams are not listed, check the ingredients list to see if any sources of saturated fat are present (see p. 35 for list). (For example, 1 gram saturated fat per slice × 9 calories per gram of fat = 9 calories from saturated fat per slice ÷ 100 calories per slice = .09 × 100 = 9% calories from saturated fat.) Remember, your goal is to get less than 30 percent of your total calories from fat and less than 10 percent of your total calories from saturated fat. Select foods with total fat calories greater than this only occasionally.

- *Ingredient listing.* Ingredients are listed in the order of greatest content. Therefore, the first few ingredients will be present in larger amounts than the ones that follow them. Beware, though: A small amount of similar ingredients can add up. For example, ingredients such as sodium nitrite (a curing agent in meats), sodium phosphate (an emulsifier found especially in processed cheese), baking soda (sodium bicarbonate), monosodium glutamate (MSG), or sodium propionate (a preservative) may be listed separately, but they can all add up to a lot of sodium.

- *Sugar (simple carbohydrate) content.* While a small amount is not harmful, sugar provides nutrient-empty calories. One teaspoon of sugar has four grams of carbohydrate and sixteen calories, with no vitamins or minerals. Most food labels do not provide the number of grams of sugar, so look for ingredients indicating the presence of sugar, such as sugar, brown sugar, honey, and high-fructose corn syrup.

• *U.S. RDA.* A suggested daily allowance for protein and certain vitamins and minerals, established by the Food and Drug Administration, the U.S. RDA provides a general labeling guideline to determine what percentage of your daily nutrient requirements is provided by one serving of the food.

• *Other label lingo.* Standards have been set for many food labeling terms. The following is a sample of some of these terms.

> Low-calorie = no more than 40 calories per serving
> Reduced-calorie = at least one-third fewer calories than a traditional product
> No added salt = no salt added in the product preparation (sodium naturally present in the food will still be there)
> Sodium-free = less than 5 milligrams of sodium per serving
> Very-low sodium = less than 35 milligrams of sodium per serving
> Low-sodium = less than 140 milligrams of sodium per serving
> Fat-free = less than 0.5 grams of fat per serving
> Low-fat = 3 grams or less of fat per serving
> Cholesterol-free = less than 2 milligrams of

cholesterol per serving and 2 grams of
saturated fat per serving
Low in cholesterol = 20 milligrams or less of
cholesterol per serving and 2 grams or less
of saturated fat per serving

On p. 46 is a sample food label. Apply the tips above in
translating the label language and testing your label know-
how.

THE SAVVY SHOPPER

Remember these guidelines when you are considering
the nutritional value of food products during your
regular excursions to the grocery store. The sample
menus on pp. 47–50 will show you how to develop a
shopping list that incorporates nutrient-packed foods high
in antioxidants, vitamins, and fiber. A sample shopping list
to go with the sample menus follows on pp. 51–57.

HONEY AND OATS BREAKFAST CEREAL

NUTRITION INFORMATION PER SERVING

SERVING SIZE   1 oz. (28g) or approximately ⅔ cup
SERVINGS PER CONTAINER   16

	Cereal	Cereal with ½ Cup Vit. A & D Fortified 2% Milk
Calories	110	180
Protein	4g	8g
Carbohydrates	21g	27g
Fiber	2g	2g
Total Fat	2g	4g
Saturated	—	2g
Unsaturated	2g	2g
Cholesterol	0mg	10mg
Sodium	160mg	220mg
Potassium	100mg	290mg

Percentage of U.S. Recommended Daily Allowances (% U.S. RDA)		
Protein	6	15
Vitamin A	30	35
Vitamin C	**	2
Thiamine	25	30
Riboflavin	20	30
Niacin	35	35
Calcium	3	16
Iron	35	35

**Contains less than 2% of the U.S. RDA for this ingredient.

Ingredients

Rolled oats, whole wheat, brown sugar, maltodextrin, partially hydrogenated vegetable oil (cottonseed and/or soybean oil), corn syrup, almonds, honey, salt, vitamin A palmitate, niacinamide, reduced iron, calcium pantothenate, thiamine, riboflavin, folic acid, sodium sulfite, natural flavors, BHT, BHA.

	Cereal	With Milk
Starch and Related Carbohydrates	15g	11g
Sucrose and Other Sugars	6g	12g
Total Carbohydrates	21g	23g

Use the sample menus as a guide, as individual nutrient requirements may vary. As you will see from the nutrient analysis of the sample menus, even when you select a healthful diet it is sometimes difficult to reach ideal nutrient levels. For example, day two the vitamin E level falls a little short, so it is especially important to take a vitamin supplement.

Daily Menus—Nutrient Totals

Day	Beta Carotene	Vitamin A	Vitamin C	Vitamin E	Dietary Fiber	Total Fat	% of Calories From Total Fat	Saturated Fat	% of Calories From Saturated Fat	Total Calories
DAY ONE	28 mg	5,761 I.U.	551 mg	33 mg	24 g	46 g	23%	12 g	6%	1,839
DAY TWO	22 mg	5,102 I.U.	345 mg	16 mg	35 g	38 g	19%	12 g	6%	1,821
DAY THREE	18 mg	4,715 I.U.	336 mg	31 mg	27 g	59 g	23%	14 g	6%	2,277

	Day 1	Day 2	Day 3
Breakfast	1 oz. dry cereal (fortified with 100% of the USRDA for select vitamins) with 1 medium banana and 1 cup 1% or nonfat (skim) milk ¾ cup orange juice coffee or tea	2 medium whole-grain waffles with 2 tsp. low-calorie syrup and 2 tsp. margarine ½ cup low-fat cottage cheese with 1 cup papaya chunks coffee or tea	3 egg white omelet with ½ cup shredded vegetables (tomatoes, peppers, carrots) with ¼ cup 1% or nonfat (skim) milk and cooked in 2 tsp. vegetable oil 2 slices whole-grain toast with 2 tsp. fruit preserves ½ cup apricot nectar coffee or tea

48

	Day 1	Day 2	Day 3
Lunch	1 toasted whole-wheat English muffin with ¼ cup tomato sauce and 3 ounces cooked, ground turkey	1 cup whole-wheat noodles with 1 cup mixed, steamed vegetables (broccoli, cauliflower, carrots) and ¼ cup tomato sauce, topped with 2 ounces low-fat cheese	3 ounces tuna with ¼ cup diced red peppers and 1 Tbs. low-fat mayonnaise
	1 cup raw vegetables (broccoli, cauliflower, tomato) with 1 Tbs. low-fat salad dressing	3 sliced apricots with ½ cup low-fat frozen yogurt with ¼ cup wheat germ topping	1 medium kaiser roll
	1 slice pumpkin bread		½ cup carrot-raisin salad
	seltzer water	1 cup vegetable juice cocktail	1 large slice watermelon
			seltzer water

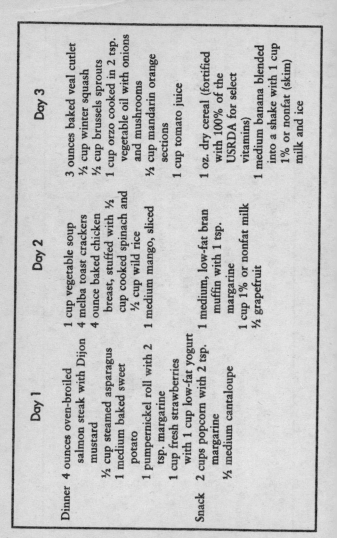

	Day 1	Day 2	Day 3
Dinner	4 ounces oven-broiled salmon steak with Dijon mustard	1 cup vegetable soup	3 ounces baked veal cutlet
	½ cup steamed asparagus	4 melba toast crackers	½ cup winter squash
	1 medium baked sweet potato	4 ounce baked chicken breast, stuffed with ½ cup cooked spinach and ½ cup wild rice	½ cup brussels sprouts
	1 pumpernickel roll with 2 tsp. margarine		1 cup orzo cooked in 2 tsp. vegetable oil with onions and mushrooms
	1 cup fresh strawberries with 1 cup low-fat yogurt	1 medium mango, sliced	½ cup mandarin orange sections
			1 cup tomato juice
Snack	2 cups popcorn with 2 tsp. margarine	1 medium, low-fat bran muffin with 1 tsp. margarine	1 oz. dry cereal (fortified with 100% of the USRDA for select vitamins)
	¼ medium cantaloupe	1 cup 1% or nonfat milk	1 medium banana blended into a shake with 1 cup 1% or nonfat (skim) milk and ice
		½ grapefruit	

SHOPPING LIST

Food Items	Beta carotene	Vitamin C	Vitamin E	Fiber	Cruciferous
FRUITS					
☐ Apricots	x	x		x	
☐ Banana		x		x	
☐ Cantaloupe	x	x		x	
☐ Mandarin oranges and grapefruit	x	x	x	x	
☐ Mangoes		x	x	x	
☐ Papaya	x	x		x	
☐ Raisins		x		x	

Food Items	Beta carotene	Vitamin C	Vitamin E	Fiber	Cruciferous
☐ Strawberries		x		x	
☐ Watermelon		x			
VEGETABLES					
☐ Asparagus		x		x	
☐ Broccoli	x	x		x	x
☐ Brussels Sprouts	x	x		x	x
☐ Cabbage		x		x	x
☐ Carrots	x			x	
☐ Cauliflower		x			x
☐ Red Pepper	x	x			
☐ Spinach	x	x			

Food Items	Beta carotene	Vitamin C	Vitamin E	Fiber	Cruciferous
STARCHY VEGETABLES					
☐ Squash, winter	x	x		x	
☐ Sweet potatoes	x	x		x	
BREADS, CEREALS, PASTA AND RICE					
☐ Fortified cereal		x		x	
☐ Breads, whole-wheat bread, pita, rolls, and English muffins				x	
☐ Melba toast					
☐ Muffins, low-fat bran				x	
☐ Noodles, whole-wheat				x	

Food Items	Beta carotene	Vitamin C	Vitamin E	Fiber	Cruciferous
☐ Orzo					
☐ Pumpkin bread	x			x	
☐ Rice, brown or wild				x	
☐ Waffles, whole-grain				x	
MEATS					
☐ Chicken, breasts					
☐ Fish, fillets (salmon, sole, swordfish)			x		
☐ Tuna, water-packed			x		

Food Items	Beta carotene	Vitamin C	Vitamin E	Fiber	Cruciferous
☐ Turkey, lean ground					
☐ Veal, cutlets					
DAIRY PRODUCTS					
☐ Cheese, low-fat cottage and mozzarella, part-skim ricotta					
☐ Eggs					
☐ Milk, 1% or nonfat					
☐ Yogurt, low-fat					
☐ Yogurt, low-fat frozen					

Food Items	Beta carotene	Vitamin C	Vitamin E	Fiber	Cruciferous
BEVERAGES					
☐ Apricot nectar	x		x		
☐ Orange juice		x			
☐ Seltzer water					
☐ Tomato juice	x	x		x	
☐ Vegetable juice cocktail	x	x		x	
MISCELLANEOUS					
☐ Margarine			x		
☐ Mayonnaise, low-fat			x		

Food Items	Beta carotene	Vitamin C	Vitamin E	Fiber	Cruciferous
☐ Mustard, Dijon					
☐ Popcorn, plain				x	
☐ Preserves, fruit					
☐ Salad dressing, low-fat			x		
☐ Syrup, low-calorie					
☐ Tomato sauce		x		x	
☐ Vegetable oil			x		
☐ Vegetable stew	x	x		x	

HOW TO USE THE FOOD TABLES

The food tables* in this book will provide you with the nutrient know-how to select a healthful diet. The foods in the tables have been categorized by the USDA's food groups. When selecting foods from the tables, remember that your own particular life-style affects your nutrient needs.

The tables provide nutrient values in both standard serving size and in grams. The milligrams of beta carotene, vitamins C and E, International Units (I.U.) of vitamin A, grams of dietary fiber, total fat and saturated fat, and number of calories are indicated for each food item. The cruciferous vegetables are identified by an asterisk (*). To help make the tables easy to use, the nutrient values have been rounded to the nearest whole number. A dash (——) in the table indicates that nutrient information was not available for that food item. When foods have only a trace (less than 0.5) of a particular nutrient, a value of "tr" is given. A portion of the vitamin A listed in the food tables is derived from the beta carotene in the foods. In the case of all fruits and vegetables, 100 percent of the vitamin A is derived from beta carotene.

*Nutrient values in this book are derived from the University of Minnesota Nutrition Coordinating Center's (NCC) Nutrient Database Version 20, release date October 1991.

5
FOOD TABLES

FRUITS AND VEGETABLES
Fruits

Food Description/ Portion	Weight (grams)	Beta Carotene (mg)	Vitamin A (I.U.)	Vitamin C (mg)	Vitamin E (mg)	Dietary Fiber (grams)	Total Fat (grams)	Saturated Fat (grams)	Calories
Apple, fresh with skin (1 medium)	138	tr	73	8	1	3	1	tr	81
Applesauce, unsweetened (½ cup)	122	tr	35	1	tr	2	tr	tr	52
Apricots, fresh (3 medium)	106	1	1,109	11	1	3	tr	tr	51
Avocado (1 small)	173	1	1,059	14	2	8	27	4	279
Banana, fresh (1 medium)	114	tr	92	10	tr	2	1	tr	105
Blackberries, fresh (1 cup)	144	tr	238	30	1	5	1	0	75
Blueberries, fresh (1 cup)	145	tr	145	19	1	2	1	0	81
Cantaloupe, fresh (½ medium)	461	8	12,688	195	1	3	1	0	161

Food Description/ Portion	Weight (grams)	Beta Carotene (mg)	Vitamin A (I.U.)	Vitamin C (mg)	Vitamin E (mg)	Dietary Fiber (grams)	Total Fat (grams)	Saturated Fat (grams)	Calories
Cherries, fresh, sweet (½ cup)	73	tr	155	5	tr	1	1	tr	52
Cranberries, fresh (1 cup)	95	tr	44	13	0	3	tr	0	47
Figs, fresh (2 medium)	100	tr	142	2	0	3	tr	tr	72
Grapes, fresh (½ cup)	80	tr	58	9	tr	1	tr	tr	57
Grapefruit, fresh (1 medium)	291	tr	361	100	1	4	tr	tr	93
Kiwi fruit, fresh (1 medium)	76	tr	133	74	1	1	tr	0	46
Lemon, fresh (1 medium)	58	tr	17	31	0	1	tr	tr	17
Mango, fresh (1 medium)	207	5	8,061	57	2	6	1	tr	135
Nectarine, fresh (1 medium)	136	tr	151	7	1	2	1	0	67
Orange, fresh (1 medium)	131	tr	269	70	tr	3	tr	tr	62

Food Description/ Portion	Weight (grams)	Beta Carotene (mg)	Vitamin A (I.U.)	Vitamin C (mg)	Vitamin E (mg)	Dietary Fiber (grams)	Total Fat (grams)	Saturated Fat (grams)	Calories
Orange, mandarin (1 medium)	84	1	773	26	0	1	tr	tr	37
Papaya, fresh (1 cup)	140	tr	398	87	0	4	tr	tr	55
Peach, fresh (1 medium)	87	tr	465	6	1	1	tr	tr	37
Pear, fresh (1 medium)	166	tr	33	7	1	6	1	tr	98
Persimmon, raw (1 medium)	168	2	3,641	13	0	3	tr	0	118
Pineapple, fresh (1 slice)	84	tr	19	13	tr	1	tr	tr	41
Plum, fresh (1 medium)	66	tr	213	6	tr	1	tr	tr	36
Pomegranate, fresh (1 medium)	154	0	0	9	0	6	tr	0	105
Raspberries, fresh (1 cup)	123	tr	160	31	1	3	1	tr	60

Food Description/ Portion	Weight (grams)	Beta Carotene (mg)	Vitamin A (I.U.)	Vitamin C (mg)	Vitamin E (mg)	Dietary Fiber (grams)	Total Fat (grams)	Saturated Fat (grams)	Calories
Rhubarb, unsweetened, stewed (1 cup)	242	tr	220	17	tr	6	0	0	12
Strawberries, fresh/frozen, unsweetened (1 cup)	149	tr	40	84	tr	2	1	tr	45
Watermelon, fresh (1 slice)	482	1	1,764	46	0	1	1	0	154
FRUIT/VEGETABLE SALADS									
Apricots, sweetened, canned, (½ cup)	129	1	1,587	4	1	2	tr	tr	107
Carrot-raisin (½ cup)	142	4	7,356	5	2	2	9	1	142

63

Food Description/ Portion	Weight (grams)	Beta Carotene (mg)	Vitamin A (I.U.)	Vitamin C (mg)	Vitamin E (mg)	Dietary Fiber (grams)	Total Fat (grams)	Saturated Fat (grams)	Calories
Mandarin orange sections, sweetened, canned (½ cup)	127	1	1,067	25	1	1	tr	tr	77
Fruit cup, fresh (1 cup)	194	tr	184	53	1	3	1	tr	99
DRIED FRUITS									
Apples, dried (½ cup)	43	0	0	2	0	4	tr	tr	105
Apple chips (½ cup)	46	0	0	9	2	4	8	1	193
Apricots, dried (½ cup)	65	3	4,706	2	1	5	tr	tr	155
Banana chips (½ cup)	46	tr	124	3	tr	3	3	2	169
Dates, dried (½ cup)	89	tr	45	0	0	4	tr	0	245

Food Description/ Portion	Weight (grams)	Beta Carotene (mg)	Vitamin A (I.U.)	Vitamin C (mg)	Vitamin E (mg)	Dietary Fiber (grams)	Total Fat (grams)	Saturated Fat (grams)	Calories
Figs, dried (½ cup)	100	tr	132	1	0	8	1	tr	254
Peaches, dried (½ cup)	80	1	1,730	4	0	6	1	tr	191
Pears, dried (½ cup)	90	tr	3	6	0	11	1	tr	236
Prunes, dried, uncooked (½ cup)	81	1	1,600	3	1	5	tr	tr	192
Raisins (¼ cup)	39	0	0	2	tr	1	tr	tr	115
FRUIT JUICES									
Apple juice, sweetened (½ cup)	124	0	0	1	tr	tr	0	0	68
Apricot nectar (½ cup)	126	1	1,652	1	1	1	tr	tr	70
Cranapple juice, sweetened (½ cup)	123	tr	4	39	0	tr	0	0	82

Food Description/ Portion	Weight (grams)	Beta Carotene (mg)	Vitamin A (I.U.)	Vitamin C (mg)	Vitamin E (mg)	Dietary Fiber (grams)	Total Fat (grams)	Saturated Fat (grams)	Calories
Cranberry juice, sweetened, (½ cup)	127	tr	5	45	0	0	tr	tr	72
Grape juice, sweetened, frozen (½ cup)	125	tr	10	30	0	tr	tr	tr	64
Grapefruit juice, sweetened, frozen/canned (½ cup)	125	0	0	34	tr	tr	tr	tr	58
Lemonade/ limeade, sweetened (½ cup)	124	tr	26	5	0	tr	tr	tr	50
Lemon juice, unsweetened, fresh/frozen (½ cup)	122	tr	18	30	tr	tr	tr	tr	26

Food Description/ Portion	Weight (grams)	Beta Carotene (mg)	Vitamin A (I.U.)	Vitamin C (mg)	Vitamin E (mg)	Dietary Fiber (grams)	Total Fat (grams)	Saturated Fat (grams)	Calories
Orange juice, sweetened, frozen/canned (½ cup)	125	tr	212	42	tr	tr	tr	tr	65
Pineapple juice, frozen/canned (½ cup)	125	tr	6	13	tr	tr	tr	0	70
Prune juice, bottled (½ cup)	128	tr	4	5	tr	1	tr	0	91
VEGETABLES									
Artichokes, cooked (½ cup)	84	tr	149	8	tr	3	tr	tr	42
Asparagus, fresh/frozen, cooked (½ cup)	90	tr	736	22	1	2	tr	tr	25

Food Description/ Portion	Weight (grams)	Beta Carotene (mg)	Vitamin A (I.U.)	Vitamin C (mg)	Vitamin E (mg)	Dietary Fiber (grams)	Total Fat (grams)	Saturated Fat (grams)	Calories
Beets, red, fresh/frozen, cooked (½ cup)	85	tr	11	5	tr	2	tr	tr	26
Broccoli, raw* (½ cup)	44	tr	561	41	tr	1	tr	tr	12
Broccoli, fresh/frozen, cooked* (½ cup)	92	1	1,740	37	1	3	tr	tr	26
Brussel sprouts, fresh/frozen, cooked* (½ cup)	78	tr	456	35	1	4	tr	tr	33
Cabbage, raw* (1 cup)	70	tr	88	33	1	1	tr	tr	17
Carrots, raw (½ cup)	55	5	8,511	5	tr	2	tr	tr	24

Food Description/ Portion	Weight (grams)	Beta Carotene (mg)	Vitamin A (I.U.)	Vitamin C (mg)	Vitamin E (mg)	Dietary Fiber (grams)	Total Fat (grams)	Saturated Fat (grams)	Calories
Carrots, canned, drained solids (½ cup)	73	6	10,055	2	tr	1	tr	tr	17
Carrots, fresh/frozen, cooked (½ cup)	78	11	19,152	2	1	2	tr	tr	35
Cauliflower, raw* (½ cup)	50	tr	8	36	tr	1	tr	tr	12
Cauliflower, fresh/frozen, cooked* (½ cup)	90	tr	20	28	tr	1	tr	tr	17
Celery, raw (½ cup)	120	tr	161	8	tr	2	tr	tr	19
Celery, fresh/frozen, cooked (½ cup)	75	tr	99	5	tr	2	tr	tr	14

Food Description/ Portion	Weight (grams)	Beta Carotene (mg)	Vitamin A (I.U.)	Vitamin C (mg)	Vitamin E (mg)	Dietary Fiber (grams)	Total Fat (grams)	Saturated Fat (grams)	Calories
Cucumber, raw (½ cup)	52	tr	23	2	tr	tr	tr	tr	7
Eggplant, cooked (½ cup)	48	tr	31	1	tr	1	tr	tr	13
Endive, raw (1 cup)	29	tr	595	2	tr	1	tr	tr	5
Garlic, fresh (1 tsp)	3	0	0	1	0	tr.	tr	0	5
Green beans, fresh, cooked (½ cup)	68	tr	356	6	tr	2	tr	tr	18
Greens, collards, fresh/frozen, cooked* (1 cup)	128	2	3,491	15	3	3	tr	0	35
Kohlrabi, fresh/frozen, cooked* (½ cup)	83	tr	29	45	0	2	tr	tr	24

Food Description/ Portion	Weight (grams)	Beta Carotene (mg)	Vitamin A (I.U.)	Vitamin C (mg)	Vitamin E (mg)	Dietary Fiber (grams)	Total Fat (grams)	Saturated Fat (grams)	Calories
Lettuce, raw (1 cup)	55	tr	182	2	tr	1	tr	tr	7
Mushrooms, raw, whole/sliced (½ cup)	35	0	0	1	tr	tr	tr	tr	9
Mushrooms, fresh/frozen, cooked (½ cup)	78	0	0	3	0	2	tr	tr	21
Mushrooms, canned, drained (½ cup)	78	0	0	0	tr	2	tr	tr	19
Okra, fresh/frozen, cooked (½ cup)	92	tr	473	11	0	4	tr	tr	34
Onions, raw (½ cup)	80	0	0	5	tr	2	tr	tr	30
Onions, fresh/frozen, cooked (½ cup)	105	0	0	6	tr	2	tr	tr	46

Food Description/ Portion	Weight (grams)	Beta Carotene (mg)	Vitamin A (I.U.)	Vitamin C (mg)	Vitamin E (mg)	Dietary Fiber (grams)	Total Fat (grams)	Saturated Fat (grams)	Calories
Pepper, green, raw (½ cup)	50	tr	316	45	tr	1	tr	tr	14
Pepper, green, fresh/frozen (½ cup)	68	tr	403	51	tr	1	tr	tr	19
Pepper, hot chili, mature red with seeds (Pequin) (1 tsp.)	2	1	1,540	tr	—	tr	tr	tr	6
Pepper, hot chili, mature red without seeds (1 tsp.)	2	1	1,917	tr	0	0	tr	tr	6
Pepper, red, raw (½ cup)	50	2	2,850	95	tr	1	tr	tr	14
Pepper, red, fresh/frozen, cooked (½ cup)	68	2	2,557	116	tr	1	tr	tr	19

Food Description/ Portion	Weight (grams)	Beta Carotene (mg)	Vitamin A (I.U.)	Vitamin C (mg)	Vitamin E (mg)	Dietary Fiber (grams)	Total Fat (grams)	Saturated Fat (grams)	Calories
Pumpkin, cooked, canned (½ cup)	123	16	27,016	5	1	1	tr	tr	42
Radish, raw* (½ cup)	58	tr	5	13	0	1	tr	tr	10
Romaine, raw (1 cup)	30	1	780	7	tr	tr	tr	tr	5
Rutabaga, fresh/frozen, cooked* (½ cup)	85	0	0	19	tr	1	tr	tr	29
Sauerkraut, canned, cooked (½ cup)	118	tr	21	17	2	4	tr	tr	22
Spinach, raw* (1 cup)	56	3	4,705	16	1	1	tr	tr	12
Spinach, fresh/frozen, cooked* (½ cup)	95	4	7,395	12	2	2	tr	tr	27

Food Description/ Portion	Weight (grams)	Beta Carotene (mg)	Vitamin A (I.U.)	Vitamin C (mg)	Vitamin E (mg)	Dietary Fiber (grams)	Total Fat (grams)	Saturated Fat (grams)	Calories
Sprouts, alfalfa, raw (1 cup)	33	tr	51	3	0	1	tr	tr	10
Squash, summer, fresh, cooked (½ cup)	90	tr	258	5	tr	1	tr	tr	18
Tomato, raw (1 cup)	180	1	1,122	34	1	1	1	tr	38
Tomato, fresh, cooked (½ cup)	120	1	892	27	2	2	1	tr	32
Tomato, canned (1 cup)	240	1	1,450	36	3	3	1	tr	48
Watercress, raw* (1 cup)	34	1	1,598	7	tr	tr	tr	—	4
Zucchini, raw (½ cup)	65	tr	221	6	tr	1	tr	tr	9
Zucchini, fresh/frozen, cooked (½ cup)	90	tr	216	4	tr	1	tr	tr	14

Food Description/ Portion	Weight (grams)	Beta Carotene (mg)	Vitamin A (I.U.)	Vitamin C (mg)	Vitamin E (mg)	Dietary Fiber (grams)	Total Fat (grams)	Saturated Fat (grams)	Calories
VEGETABLE JUICES									
Carrot juice (1 cup)	246	38	63,347	21	1	2	tr	tr	98
Tomato juice (1 cup)	243	1	1,349	44	0	2	tr	tr	41
Vegetable juice cocktail (1 cup)	242	2	2,831	67	0	2	tr	tr	46
STARCHY VEGETABLES, BREADS, CEREALS AND PASTA									
STARCHY VEGETABLES									
Beans, kidney, canned, cooked (½ cup)	89	0	0	1	tr	7	tr	tr	112
Beans, lima, dry/canned, cooked (½ cup)	94	0	0	0	tr	7	tr	tr	108

75

Food Description/ Portion	Weight (grams)	Beta Carotene (mg)	Vitamin A (I.U.)	Vitamin C (mg)	Vitamin E (mg)	Dietary Fiber (grams)	Total Fat (grams)	Saturated Fat (grams)	Calories
Beans, navy, dry/canned, cooked (½ cup)	91	tr	2	1	tr	6	1	tr	129
Beans, pinto, dry/canned, cooked (½ cup)	86	tr	2	2	tr	6	tr	tr	117
Chick-peas, dry/cooked, canned (½ cup)	82	tr	22	1	tr	4	2	tr	134
Corn, ear, cooked (1 medium)	77	tr	167	5	tr	2	1	tr	83
Corn, whole kernel, fresh/frozen, cooked (½ cup)	82	tr	204	2	tr	3	tr	tr	67
Lentils, dry/cooked, canned (½ cup)	99	tr	8	1	tr	5	tr	tr	115
Peas, black-eyed, fresh, cooked (½ cup)	83	tr	653	2	0	3	tr	tr	80

Food Description/ Portion	Weight (grams)	Beta Carotene (mg)	Vitamin A (I.U.)	Vitamin C (mg)	Vitamin E (mg)	Dietary Fiber (grams)	Total Fat (grams)	Saturated Fat (grams)	Calories
Peas, black-eyed, dry, cooked, canned (½ cup)	86	tr	13	tr	0	8	1	tr	99
Peas, Green, fresh/frozen (½ cup)	80	tr	534	8	tr	4	tr	tr	62
Peas, split, dry, cooked, canned (½ cup)	98	tr	7	tr	tr	3	tr	tr	116
Peas and carrots, cooked, fresh/frozen (½ cup)	80	4	6,209	6	tr	3	tr	tr	38
Mixed vegetables (corn, lima beans, peas, carrots, snap beans) cooked, fresh/frozen (½ cup)	91	2	3,892	3	tr	3	tr	tr	54
Potato, baked (½ cup)	78	0	0	6	tr	1	tr	tr	67

Food Description/ Portion	Weight (grams)	Beta Carotene (mg)	Vitamin A (I.U.)	Vitamin C (mg)	Vitamin E (mg)	Dietary Fiber (grams)	Total Fat (grams)	Saturated Fat (grams)	Calories
Potato, baked, boiled with skin (1 large potato)	156	0	0	20	tr	3	tr	tr	170
Squash, winter, fresh, cooked (½ cup)	123	3	4,357	12	tr	3	1	tr	48
Sweet potato, cooked, fresh/frozen with skin (1 small)	128	17	27,823	31	1	3	tr	tr	131
Sweet potato, cooked, fresh/frozen (½ cup)	78	17	27,823	32	1	3	tr	tr	132
Sweet potato, canned, drained solids (½ cup)	100	5	7,983	26	tr	1	tr	tr	91
Sweet potatoes, candied (1 medium)	142	15	25,197	28	1	3	6	1	241

Food Description/Portion	Weight (grams)	Beta Carotene (mg)	Vitamin A (I.U.)	Vitamin C (mg)	Vitamin E (mg)	Dietary Fiber (grams)	Total Fat (grams)	Saturated Fat (grams)	Calories
BAGELS									
Bagel, egg (1 medium)	55	tr	18	0	tr	1	3	tr	165
Bagel, oat bran (1 medium)	55	tr	5	0	tr	2	1	tr	141
Bagel, plain (1 medium)	55	0	0	0	tr	1	2	tr	165
Bagel, rye (1 medium)	66	0	0	0	tr	3	1	tr	176
Bagel, whole wheat (1 medium)	55	0	0	0	tr	4	1	tr	153
BREAKFAST BREADS									
French toast (1 medium)	43	tr	58	tr	tr	tr	2	1	95
Pancake, homemade (2 medium)	21	tr	28	tr	tr	tr	2	1	54

Food Description/ Portion	Weight (grams)	Beta Carotene (mg)	Vitamin A (I.U.)	Vitamin C (mg)	Vitamin E (mg)	Dietary Fiber (grams)	Total Fat (grams)	Saturated Fat (grams)	Calories
Pancake, from mix with water (2 medium)	21	tr	61	tr	tr	1	1	tr	74
Pancake, from mix with egg, milk, oil (2 medium)	21	tr	90	tr	tr	tr	2	1	82
Waffle, frozen (2 large)	34	tr	38	tr	tr	tr	2	tr	67
MUFFINS									
Bran, homemade (1 medium)	50	tr	22	tr	tr	2	2	1	99
Carrot, homemade/ commercial (1 medium)	58	1	2,143	1	1	1	6	3	175

Food Description/ Portion	Weight (grams)	Beta Carotene (mg)	Vitamin A (I.U.)	Vitamin C (mg)	Vitamin E (mg)	Dietary Fiber (grams)	Total Fat (grams)	Saturated Fat (grams)	Calories
Corn, homemade/ commercial (1 medium)	40	tr	89	tr	1	1	4	2	110
English muffin, all except whole wheat (1 medium)	57	0	0	0	tr	2	1	tr	134
English muffin, whole wheat (1 medium)	57	tr	17	tr	1	2	3	tr	145
Oat bran/oatmeal, homemade (1 medium)	47	tr	59	tr	1	1	6	3	142
Pumpkin, homemade (1 medium)	58	2	3,418	1	1	1	4	2	178
ROLLS									
Croissant (1 medium)	55	tr	401	tr	tr	1	12	7	172

Food Description/ Portion	Weight (grams)	Beta Carotene (mg)	Vitamin A (I.U.)	Vitamin C (mg)	Vitamin E (mg)	Dietary Fiber (grams)	Total Fat (grams)	Saturated Fat (grams)	Calories
Hamburger roll (1 medium)	43	0	0	0	tr	1	2	1	129
Hotdog roll (1 medium)	43	0	0	0	tr	1	2	1	129
Kaiser roll (1 medium)	50	0	0	0	tr	2	2	tr	156
Roll, rye (1 medium)	36	0	0	0	tr	2	1	tr	94
Roll, white, dinner (1 medium)	36	0	0	0	tr	1	2	1	107
SLICED BREADS									
Bread, corn (1 slice)	59	tr	132	tr	1	1	8	3	195
Bread, egg (2 slices)	65	tr	80	0	tr	2	3	1	189
Bread, Italian (2 slices)	60	0	0	0	tr	2	1	tr	166

Food Description/ Portion	Weight (grams)	Beta Carotene (mg)	Vitamin A (I.U.)	Vitamin C (mg)	Vitamin E (mg)	Dietary Fiber (grams)	Total Fat (grams)	Saturated Fat (grams)	Calories
Bread, nut (1 slice)	58	tr	47	tr	1	1	7	1	182
Bread, oatmeal (2 slices)	60	tr	14	tr	1	2	4	1	166
Bread, pumpkin, without nuts (1 slice)	45	2	3,418	1	1	1	5	2	163
Bread, raisin (2 slices)	45	0	0	0	tr	2	1	tr	118
Bread, rye (2 slices)	57	0	0	0	tr	4	2	tr	150
Bread, white (2 slices)	50	0	0	0	tr	1	2	tr	135
Bread, whole-wheat, mixed-grain, wheat-germ, granola (2 slices)	57	0	0	0	tr	3	2	tr	139

Food Description/ Portion	Weight (grams)	Beta Carotene (mg)	Vitamin A (I.U.)	Vitamin C (mg)	Vitamin E (mg)	Dietary Fiber (grams)	Total Fat (grams)	Saturated Fat (grams)	Calories
OTHER									
Tortilla, corn, plain (1 medium)	21	tr	36	0	tr	1	1	tr	48
Tortilla, taco shell (1 medium)	13	tr	55	0	tr	1	3	1	59
CEREALS, READY-TO-EAT									

Many dry cereals are fortified with 25% of the U.S. RDA, and a few dry cereals are fortified with 100% of the U.S. RDA (e.g., Product 19, Total) for select vitamins (e.g., vitamins A & C) per serving. Check your cereal label.

Bran flakes (½ cup)	28	0	0	27	tr	9	1	tr	71
Corn flakes (½ cup)	28	0	750	15	tr	tr	tr	tr	110
Granola, with soybean oil (¼ cup)	28	0	0	0	1	2	5	1	131

Food Description/ Portion	Weight (grams)	Beta Carotene (mg)	Vitamin A (I.U.)	Vitamin C (mg)	Vitamin E (mg)	Dietary Fiber (grams)	Total Fat (grams)	Saturated Fat (grams)	Calories
Grape-Nuts®, Post (¾ cup)	28	0	1,235	0	tr	3	tr	tr	104
Product 19®, Kellogg's (1 cup)	28	0	750	60	20	1	tr	tr	108
Total®, General Mills (¾ cup)	28	0	4,938	59	20	3	1	tr	99
Wheat germ (¼ cup)	28	0	0	2	5	4	3	1	109
Wheaties®, General Mills (1 cup)	28	0	1,252	15	tr	2	tr	tr	99
CEREALS, COOKED									
Cream of rice (1 cup)	244	0	0	0	tr	1	tr	tr	140
Cream of wheat (1 cup)	251	0	0	0	tr	1	1	tr	134
Oat bran (1 cup)	219	tr	37	0	tr	5	3	1	90

Food Description/Portion	Weight (grams)	Beta Carotene (mg)	Vitamin A (I.U.)	Vitamin C (mg)	Vitamin E (mg)	Dietary Fiber (grams)	Total Fat (grams)	Saturated Fat (grams)	Calories
Oatmeal (1 cup)	234	tr	38	0	1	4	2	tr	145
CRACKERS									
Breadsticks, plain (1 medium)	10	0	0	0	0	tr	tr	tr	28
Graham crackers (4 pieces)	14	tr	tr	0	tr	tr	1	1	58
Matzos (1 board)	28	0	0	0	tr	1	tr	tr	111
Melba toast (4 pieces)	14	0	0	0	0	tr	tr	tr	51
Saltines (4 pieces)	14	0	0	0	tr	tr	2	1	61
Triscuit (4 pieces)	14	0	0	0	tr	1	2	tr	58
Zwieback (4 pieces)	14	tr	8	tr	tr	tr	1	1	60

PASTA AND RICE

Food Description/ Portion	Weight (grams)	Beta Carotene (mg)	Vitamin A (I.U.)	Vitamin C (mg)	Vitamin E (mg)	Dietary Fiber (grams)	Total Fat (grams)	Saturated Fat (grams)	Calories
Macaroni, white, cooked (1 cup)	140	0	0	0	tr	1	1	tr	197
Macaroni, whole-wheat, cooked (1 cup)	140	0	0	0	tr	4	1	tr	174
Noodles, chow mein (1 cup)	45	tr	38	0	2	2	14	2	237
Noodles, egg, cooked (½ cup)	160	tr	32	0	tr	3	2	1	213
Rice, brown, cooked (1 cup)	195	0	0	0	1	3	2	tr	216
Rice, white, cooked, (1 cup)	205	0	0	0	tr	1	1	tr	264

MILK PRODUCTS
MILKS

Food Description/ Portion	Weight (grams)	Beta Carotene (mg)	Vitamin A (I.U.)	Vitamin C (mg)	Vitamin E (mg)	Dietary Fiber (grams)	Total Fat (grams)	Saturated Fat (grams)	Calories
Buttermilk, whole (1 cup)	240	tr	336	2	tr	0	8	5	149
Buttermilk, 1% fat (1 cup)	245	tr	81	2	tr	0	2	1	99
Milk, canned, condensed, sweet (¼ cup)	77	tr	251	2	tr	0	7	4	245
Milk, canned, evaporated skim, undiluted (½ cup)	128	tr	502	2	0	0	tr	tr	100
Milk, canned, evaporated whole, undiluted (½ cup)	126	tr	306	2	tr	0	10	6	169
Milk, chocolate, whole (1 cup)	250	tr	303	2	tr	2	8	5	208

Food Description/ Portion	Weight (grams)	Beta Carotene (mg)	Vitamin A (I.U.)	Vitamin C (mg)	Vitamin E (mg)	Dietary Fiber (grams)	Total Fat (grams)	Saturated Fat (grams)	Calories
Milk, nonfat, instant, powdered (1 Tbsp.)	4	tr	101	tr	0	0	tr	tr	15
Milk, skim/nonfat (1 cup)	245	tr	500	2	0	0	tr	tr	86
Milk, whole (1 cup)	244	tr	307	2	tr	0	8	5	150
Milk, 1% fat (1 cup)	244	tr	500	2	tr	0	3	2	102
Milk, 2% fat (1 cup)	244	tr	500	2	tr	0	5	3	121
YOGURT									
Yogurt, low-fat, plain/unflavored (1 cup)	245	tr	17	2	0	0	tr	tr	137
Yogurt, vanilla, fruit, whole (1 cup)	245	tr	311	2	tr	0	8	5	292

Food Description/ Portion	Weight (grams)	Beta Carotene (mg)	Vitamin A (I.U.)	Vitamin C (mg)	Vitamin E (mg)	Dietary Fiber (grams)	Total Fat (grams)	Saturated Fat (grams)	Calories
Yogurt, low-fat, vanilla or coffee (1 cup)	245	tr	862	2	0	0	tr	tr	162
FROZEN DESSERTS									
Ice cream, light, 7% fat, vanilla (½ cup)	61	tr	174	tr	tr	0	5	3	104
Ice cream, average, 10% fat, vanilla (½ cup)	67	tr	271	tr	tr	0	7	5	135
Ice cream, rich, 16% fat, vanilla (½ cup)	74	tr	448	tr	tr	0	12	7	175
Ice milk, hardened, 5% fat, vanilla (½ cup)	66	tr	107	tr	tr	0	3	2	92

Food Description/ Portion	Weight (grams)	Beta Carotene (mg)	Vitamin A (I.U.)	Vitamin C (mg)	Vitamin E (mg)	Dietary Fiber (grams)	Total Fat (grams)	Saturated Fat (grams)	Calories
Ice milk, soft serve, 3% fat, vanilla (½ cup)	88	tr	96	1	tr	0	2	1	112
Sherbet (½ cup)	97	tr	93	2	tr	0	2	1	135
Yogurt, regular frozen vanilla (½ cup)	123	tr	156	1	tr	0	4	3	146
Yogurt, low-fat, frozen vanilla (½ cup)	123	tr	431	1	0	0	tr	tr	81

CREAM, NONDAIRY CREAMERS, AND TOPPERS

Food Description/ Portion	Weight (grams)	Beta Carotene (mg)	Vitamin A (I.U.)	Vitamin C (mg)	Vitamin E (mg)	Dietary Fiber (grams)	Total Fat (grams)	Saturated Fat (grams)	Calories
Cream, heavy whipping, (2 Tbs.)	30	tr	437	tr	tr	0	11	7	103
Cream, whipping, (2 Tbs.)	30	tr	337	tr	tr	0	9	6	87

Food Description/ Portion	Weight (grams)	Beta Carotene (mg)	Vitamin A (I.U.)	Vitamin C (mg)	Vitamin E (mg)	Dietary Fiber (grams)	Total Fat (grams)	Saturated Fat (grams)	Calories
Half-and-half cream, (2 Tbs.)	30	tr	131	tr	tr	0	3	2	39
Sour cream, low-fat, (2 Tbs.)	31	tr	200	tr	tr	0	2	1	40
Whipped topping, aerosol (2 Tbs.)	9	tr	41	0	0	tr	2	2	23
			CHEESES						
American, processed (1 ounce)	28	tr	343	0	tr	0	9	6	106
Camembert, Brie, Jarlsberg (1 ounce)	28	tr	262	0	tr	0	7	4	85
Cheddar, Colby (1 ounce)	28	tr	300	0	tr	0	9	6	114
Cheese spread (1 Tbs.)	16	tr	136	0	tr	0	4	2	49

Food Description/ Portion	Weight (grams)	Beta Carotene (mg)	Vitamin A (I.U.)	Vitamin C (mg)	Vitamin E (mg)	Dietary Fiber (grams)	Total Fat (grams)	Saturated Fat (grams)	Calories
Cottage cheese, 2% fat (½ cup)	113	tr	79	0	tr	0	2	1	101
Cottage cheese, 4% Fat (½ cup)	105	tr	171	0	tr	0	5	3	109
Cream cheese, light (2 Tbs.)	29	tr	220	0	tr	0	5	3	64
Cream, Neufchatel (1 ounce)	28	tr	318	0	tr	0	7	4	72
Edam, Gouda, Romano, Provolone (1 ounce)	28	tr	260	0	tr	0	8	5	101
Feta cheese (1 ounce)	28	tr	127	0	tr	0	6	4	75
Limburger, Bleu, Roquefort (1 ounce)	28	tr	204	0	tr	0	8	5	100
Mozzarella, part skim milk (1 ounce)	28	tr	178	0	tr	0	5	3	79

Food Description/ Portion	Weight (grams)	Beta Carotene (mg)	Vitamin A (I.U.)	Vitamin C (mg)	Vitamin E (mg)	Dietary Fiber (grams)	Total Fat (grams)	Saturated Fat (grams)	Calories
Mozzarella, whole milk (1 ounce)	28	tr	256	0	tr	0	7	4	90
Muenster, Brick, Monterey, Port Du Salut, Fontina, Cheshire (1 ounce)	28	tr	318	0	tr	0	9	5	104
Ricotta, part skim (1 ounce)	28	tr	121	0	tr	0	2	1	39
Ricotta, whole milk (1 ounce)	28	tr	138	0	tr	0	4	2	49
Swiss, Gruyere (1 ounce)	28	tr	240	0	tr	0	8	5	107

MEAT AND MEAT PRODUCTS
CHICKEN

Food Description/ Portion	Weight (grams)	Beta Carotene (mg)	Vitamin A (I.U.)	Vitamin C (mg)	Vitamin E (mg)	Dietary Fiber (grams)	Total Fat (grams)	Saturated Fat (grams)	Calories
Dark meat with skin, cooked (3 ounces)	85	tr	85	0	1	0	12	3	202

Food Description/ Portion	Weight (grams)	Beta Carotene (mg)	Vitamin A (I.U.)	Vitamin C (mg)	Vitamin E (mg)	Dietary Fiber (grams)	Total Fat (grams)	Saturated Fat (grams)	Calories
Dark meat without skin, cooked (3 ounces)	85	tr	31	0	1	0	7	2	167
Light meat with skin, cooked (3 ounces)	85	tr	47	0	tr	0	8	2	178
Light meat without skin, cooked (3 ounces)	85	tr	12	0	tr	0	3	1	140
TURKEY									
Turkey, Cornish hen, light/dark meat with skin (3 ounces)	85	tr	66	0	tr	0	10	3	190
Turkey, Cornish hen, light/dark meat without skin (3 ounces)	85	tr	21	0	tr	0	5	2	154

Food Description/ Portion	Weight (grams)	Beta Carotene (mg)	Vitamin A (I.U.)	Vitamin C (mg)	Vitamin E (mg)	Dietary Fiber (grams)	Total Fat (grams)	Saturated Fat (grams)	Calories
DUCK									
Domestic without skin, cooked (3 ounces)	85	0	65	0	tr	0	10	4	187
FISH									
Abalone, cooked, canned (3 ounces)	85	tr	4	2	tr	0	tr	tr	91
Clams, cooked, canned (1 ounce)	28	tr	157	6	tr	0	1	tr	41
Crabmeat, canned (3 ounces)	85	tr	4	2	1	0	1	tr	84
Crab, all types, fresh/frozen (3 ounces)	85	tr	5	3	1	0	2	tr	87
Gefilte fish (1 piece)	70	1	1,519	2	tr	1	2	tr	61

Food Description/ Portion	Weight (grams)	Beta Carotene (mg)	Vitamin A (I.U.)	Vitamin C (mg)	Vitamin E (mg)	Dietary Fiber (grams)	Total Fat (grams)	Saturated Fat (grams)	Calories
Haddock, smoked (3 ounces)	85	tr	62	0	tr	0	1	tr	99
Herring, canned/smoked (2 medium pieces)	80	tr	102	1	2	0	10	2	174
Salmon, pink, canned (½ cup)	89	tr	49	0	1	0	5	1	123
Sardines, canned, drained (7 medium)	84	tr	188	0	1	0	10	1	175
Shrimp, cooked, canned (3 ounces)	85	tr	186	2	2	0	1	tr	84
Scallops, cooked (3 ounces)	85	tr	144	0	1	0	1	tr	98
Tuna, canned, oil pack, drained (½ cup)	80	tr	62	0	1	0	7	1	158
Tuna, canned, water pack, drained (½ cup)	80	tr	62	0	tr	0	tr	tr	105

Food Description/ Portion	Weight (grams)	Beta Carotene (mg)	Vitamin A (I.U.)	Vitamin C (mg)	Vitamin E (mg)	Dietary Fiber (grams)	Total Fat (grams)	Saturated Fat (grams)	Calories
BEEF									
Arm roast, arm steak (3 ounces)	85	0	0	0	tr	0	8	3	176
Bottom round, roast steak with chuck roast, steak, filet mignon (3 ounces)	85	0	0	0	tr	0	8	3	176
Eye of round (3 ounces)	85	0	0	0	tr	0	4	1	153
Ground beef, hamburger, 15% fat untrimmed (3 ounces)	85	0	0	0	tr	0	17	7	244
Liver (3 ounces)	85	2	30,345	20	1	0	4	2	137
London broil, untrimmed (3 ounces)	85	0	0	0	tr	0	13	5	211

Food Description/ Portion	Weight (grams)	Beta Carotene (mg)	Vitamin A (I.U.)	Vitamin C (mg)	Vitamin E (mg)	Dietary Fiber (grams)	Total Fat (grams)	Saturated Fat (grams)	Calories
Pot roast (moist heat) (3 ounces)	85	0	0	0	tr	0	8	3	176
Prime rib, rib roast, rib steak, roast beef, (dry heat) (3 ounces)	85	0	0	0	tr	0	13	5	211
Shank (3 ounces)	85	0	0	0	tr	0	4	1	153
Sirloin steak, shell steak, T-bone steak, loin steak (3 ounces)	85	0	0	0	tr	0	8	3	176
VEAL									
Average, trimmed, cooked (3 ounces)	85	0	0	0	tr	0	5	2	139
Liver, cooked (3 ounces)	85	1	22,863	26	tr	0	6	2	140

Food Description/ Portion	Weight (grams)	Beta Carotene (mg)	Vitamin A (I.U.)	Vitamin C (mg)	Vitamin E (mg)	Dietary Fiber (grams)	Total Fat (grams)	Saturated Fat (grams)	Calories
LAMB									
Average, trimmed (3 ounces)	85	0	0	0	tr	0	8	3	173
Liver, cooked (3 ounces)	85	1	21,216	3	1	0	8	3	187
Rack, ribs, rib roast (3 ounces)	85	0	0	0	tr	0	11	4	197
PORK									
Bacon, Canadian style (2 slices)	42	0	0	9	tr	0	4	1	78
Bacon, regular, cooked (3 slices)	19	0	0	6	tr	0	9	3	73
Chop, loin, rib, sirloin, top loin, cutlet, cooked (3 ounces)	85	0	6	tr	tr	0	12	4	204

Food Description/ Portion	Weight (grams)	Beta Carotene (mg)	Vitamin A (I.U.)	Vitamin C (mg)	Vitamin E (mg)	Dietary Fiber (grams)	Total Fat (grams)	Saturated Fat (grams)	Calories
Fresh, arm picnic, roast, steak, cooked (3 ounces)	85	0	6	tr	tr	0	12	4	204
Ham (canned regular), Prosciutto, Virginia, (3 ounces)	85	0	0	19	tr	0	8	3	151
Ham, fresh (3 ounces)	85	0	8	tr	tr	0	9	3	188
Liver, cooked (3 ounces)	85	1	15,306	20	tr	0	4	1	140
LUNCHEON MEATS									
Bologna, (beef/pork) (3 ounces)	85	0	0	18	tr	0	24	9	269
Bologna (turkey/chicken) (3 ounces)	85	0	0	0	tr	0	12	4	168
Chicken breast (3 ounces)	85	tr	11	0	tr	tr	3	1	91

Food Description/ Portion	Weight (grams)	Beta Carotene (mg)	Vitamin A (I.U.)	Vitamin C (mg)	Vitamin E (mg)	Dietary Fiber (grams)	Total Fat (grams)	Saturated Fat (grams)	Calories
Corned beef, canned (3 ounces)	85	0	0	1	tr	0	13	5	213
Frankfurter (beef and pork) (1 regular)	45	0	0	12	tr	0	13	5	144
Frankfurter (chicken) (1 regular)	45	0	0	0	tr	0	8	3	102
Pastrami (beef) (3 ounces)	85	0	0	3	1	0	25	9	297
Pastrami (turkey) (3 ounces)	85	0	0	0	tr	0	5	2	120
Salami (beef and pork) (3 ounces)	85	0	0	10	tr	0	17	7	212
Turkey Breast (3 ounces)	85	tr	8	0	tr	0	2	1	97
SAUSAGES									
Italian (1 link)	50	0	0	1	tr	0	13	4	160

Food Description/ Portion	Weight (grams)	Beta Carotene (mg)	Vitamin A (I.U.)	Vitamin C (mg)	Vitamin E (mg)	Dietary Fiber (grams)	Total Fat (grams)	Saturated Fat (grams)	Calories
Knockwurst, bratwurst (1 link)	68	0	0	18	tr	0	19	7	209
Pork, fresh, cooked (3 links)	39	0	0	tr	tr	0	12	4	144
Turkey, fresh, cooked (2 links)	48	tr	39	0	tr	0	5	2	93
EGGS									
Egg, whole, raw (1 large)	50	tr	318	0	tr	0	5	2	75
Egg, white, raw (1 large)	33	0	0	0	0	0	0	0	17
Egg, yolk, raw (1 large)	17	tr	323	0	tr	0	5	2	59
Egg, scrambled with whole milk (1 large)	128	tr	1,087	tr	2	0	19	5	235

Food Description/ Portion	Weight (grams)	Beta Carotene (mg)	Vitamin A (I.U.)	Vitamin C (mg)	Vitamin E (mg)	Dietary Fiber (grams)	Total Fat (grams)	Saturated Fat (grams)	Calories
Egg substitute (Egg Beaters), prepared as directed (¼ cup)	53	tr	574	tr	tr	tr	4	1	61
Omelet, plain (1 large)	128	tr	1,087	tr	2	0	19	5	235
FAST FOODS AND PREPARED FOODS									
Baked beans with franks, canned (1 cup)	257	tr	248	17	1	9	14	5	365
Burrito, bean (1 piece)	105	tr	161	11	tr	4	4	2	183
Burrito, beef (1 piece)	163	1	1,105	7	1	2	23	9	423
Chicken salad with mayonnaise dressing (¼ cup)	53	tr	42	1	2	tr	11	2	136

Food Description/ Portion	Weight (grams)	Beta Carotene (mg)	Vitamin A (I.U.)	Vitamin C (mg)	Vitamin E (mg)	Dietary Fiber (grams)	Total Fat (grams)	Saturated Fat (grams)	Calories
Chili con carne with beans, homemade/ commercial (1 cup)	255	1	1,181	29	2	7	13	5	282
Egg roll, shrimp and pork (1 piece)	101	tr	90	3	2	1	11	3	158
Egg salad with mayonnaise (¼ cup)	56	tr	260	1	1	tr	8	2	103
Falafel (1 piece)	31	tr	33	tr	1	1	5	1	75
Fish sticks, breaded, commercial (3 ounces)	85	tr	11	0	1	1	8	1	196
French fried potatoes (1 ounce)	28	0	0	3	1	1	5	2	85
Hash browns (1 ounce)	28	0	0	2	1	tr	4	1	58

Food Description/ Portion	Weight (grams)	Beta Carotene (mg)	Vitamin A (I.U.)	Vitamin C (mg)	Vitamin E (mg)	Dietary Fiber (grams)	Total Fat (grams)	Saturated Fat (grams)	Calories
Lo mein, pork (½ cup)	80	tr	72	tr	1	tr	4	1	93
Macaroni and cheese, prepared from packaged mix (½ cup)	105	tr	495	tr	1	1	9	2	200
Pizza rolls (2 pieces)	28	tr	104	2	tr	tr	4	1	82
Pizza, cheese, thin crust/french bread, frozen (1 slice)	71	tr	390	3	tr	1	5	3	171
Ravioli, meat, canned (1 cup)	223	1	1,314	2	tr	3	7	4	240
Submarine sandwich, bologna, salami, and cheese (1 sandwich)	153	tr	276	8	1	2	22	9	435
Taco, bean (1 medium)	89	tr	251	1	tr	4	13	6	220

Food Description/Portion	Weight (grams)	Beta Carotene (mg)	Vitamin A (I.U.)	Vitamin C (mg)	Vitamin E (mg)	Dietary Fiber (grams)	Total Fat (grams)	Saturated Fat (grams)	Calories
Taco, beef (1 medium)	91	tr	617	2	1	1	16	8	253
Tuna salad with mayonnaise (¾ cup)	50	tr	51	1	1	tr	8	1	113
SOUPS AND STEWS									
Bean soup, canned, diluted (1 cup)	250	1	878	2	tr	4	6	2	170
Beef broth, bouillon, canned, diluted (1 cup)	243	0	0	1	0	tr	0	0	29
Beef vegetable stew (1 cup)	245	7	11,556	7	1	3	23	9	369
Borscht, beet, without sour cream (1 cup)	244	2	3,817	10	1	3	3	1	83

Food Description/ Portion	Weight (grams)	Beta Carotene (mg)	Vitamin A (I.U.)	Vitamin C (mg)	Vitamin E (mg)	Dietary Fiber (grams)	Total Fat (grams)	Saturated Fat (grams)	Calories
Beef stew, canned, ready to serve, vegetable varieties (1 cup)	240	4	5,878	6	1	2	4	1	122
Ready to serve, canned, meat/poultry varieties, with vegetables or noodles (1 cup)	240	2	2,611	7	1	2	5	3	170
Chicken broth, bouillon, canned, diluted (1 cup)	243	0	0	1	0	tr	1	tr	24
Chicken vegetable, with noodle, homemade (1 cup)	240	tr	359	7	1	2	4	1	167

Food Description/ Portion	Weight (grams)	Beta Carotene (mg)	Vitamin A (I.U.)	Vitamin C (mg)	Vitamin E (mg)	Dietary Fiber (grams)	Total Fat (grams)	Saturated Fat (grams)	Calories
Chicken vegetable stew, light, dark meat without skin, with vegetables (1 cup)	245	5	8,257	5	1	2	6	2	193
Chowder, clam/Manhattan, canned, undiluted (1 cup)	251	1	1,925	8	1	2	4	1	153
Cream of mushroom, canned, undiluted (1 cup)	251	0	0	2	7	1	19	5	259
Cream of pea, canned, undiluted (1 cup)	263	tr	402	3	tr	6	6	3	329
Gazpacho, homemade (1 cup)	255	tr	623	31	3	1	17	3	191
Minestrone (1 cup)	244	1	1,113	0	tr	tr	4	1	95

Food Description/ Portion	Weight (grams)	Beta Carotene (mg)	Vitamin A (I.U.)	Vitamin C (mg)	Vitamin E (mg)	Dietary Fiber (grams)	Total Fat (grams)	Saturated Fat (grams)	Calories
Tomato soup, canned, undiluted (1 cup)	251	1	1,393	133	tr	3	4	1	171
Vegetable stew, without meat (1 cup)	245	9	15,717	10	1	4	4	1	160
SAUCES AND GRAVIES									
Gravy, au jus (¼ cup)	63	0	0	1	0	0	tr	tr	10
Barbecue sauce, bottled (1 Tbs.)	16	tr	136	1	0	tr	tr	tr	12
Duck sauce (1 Tbs.)	14	tr	74	2	tr	tr	tr	0	16
Gravy, meat, prepared with water (¼ cup)	59	0	0	tr	tr	tr	4	2	60

Food Description/ Portion	Weight (grams)	Beta Carotene (mg)	Vitamin A (I.U.)	Vitamin C (mg)	Vitamin E (mg)	Dietary Fiber (grams)	Total Fat (grams)	Saturated Fat (grams)	Calories
Gravy, poultry, prepared with water (¼ cup)	48	tr	397	tr	tr	tr	1	tr	31
Hollandaise, canned (1 Tbs.)	16	tr	145	tr	tr	tr	4	3	44
Italian, without meat, canned (½ cup)	120	tr	750	6	1	3	5	1	84
Pesto (1 Tbs.)	8	tr	51	tr	1	tr	6	1	54
Tomato paste, canned (¼ cup)	66	1	1,617	28	0	3	1	tr	55
Tomato sauce, without fat, canned (½ cup)	123	tr	1,199	16	0	2	tr	tr	37
White clam sauce (¼ cup)	50	tr	310	5	1	tr	3	1	61

Food Description/ Portion	Weight (grams)	Beta Carotene (mg)	Vitamin A (I.U.)	Vitamin C (mg)	Vitamin E (mg)	Dietary Fiber (grams)	Total Fat (grams)	Saturated Fat (grams)	Calories
OTHER									
Paprika (1 tsp.)	2	1	1,273	1	—	tr	tr	tr	6
Chili powder (1 tsp.)	3	1	908	2	—	1	tr	tr	8
FATS AND OILS									
OILS									
Canola (1 Tbs.)	14	0	0	0	3	0	14	1	120
Corn (1 Tbs.)	14	0	0	0	3	0	14	2	120
Olive (1 Tbs.)	14	0	0	0	2	0	14	2	119
Peanut (1 Tbs.)	14	0	0	0	2	0	14	2	119
Safflower (1 Tbs.)	14	0	0	0	5	0	14	1	120

Food Description/Portion	Weight (grams)	Beta Carotene (mg)	Vitamin A (I.U.)	Vitamin C (mg)	Vitamin E (mg)	Dietary Fiber (grams)	Total Fat (grams)	Saturated Fat (grams)	Calories
Soybean, partially hydrogenated (1 Tbs.)	14	0	0	0	2	0	14	2	120
Sunflower (1 Tbs.)	14	0	0	0	8	0	14	1	120
MARGARINE									
Corn, diet (1 tsp.)	5	tr	247	0	1	0	2	tr	17
Corn, stick/rub (1 tsp.)	5	tr	207	tr	1	0	4	1	34
Soybean, diet (1 tsp.)	5	tr	247	0	tr	0	2	tr	17
Soybean, stick/rub (1 tsp.)	5	tr	155	tr	tr	0	4	1	34
Safflower, stick/rub (1 tsp.)	5	tr	207	tr	tr	0	4	1	34
Sunflower, diet (1 tsp.)	5	tr	247	0	1	0	2	tr	17

Food Description/ Portion	Weight (grams)	Beta Carotene (mg)	Vitamin A (I.U.)	Vitamin C (mg)	Vitamin E (mg)	Dietary Fiber (grams)	Total Fat (grams)	Saturated Fat (grams)	Calories
Sunflower, stick/tub									
(1 tsp.)	5	tr	207	tr	1	0	4	1	34
SPREADS									
Corn									
(1 tsp.)	5	tr	229	tr	1	0	3	1	26
Soybean									
(1 tsp.)	5	tr	218	0	1	0	3	1	31
Sunflower									
(1 tsp.)	5	tr	218	0	1	0	3	1	31
NUTS									
Almonds									
(¼ cup)	36	0	0	tr	6	3	19	2	209
Brazil nuts									
(¼ cup)	35	0	0	tr	3	2	23	6	230
Cashews									
(¼ cup)	33	0	0	0	1	2	16	3	187

Food Description/ Portion	Weight (grams)	Beta Carotene (mg)	Vitamin A (I.U.)	Vitamin C (mg)	Vitamin E (mg)	Dietary Fiber (grams)	Total Fat (grams)	Saturated Fat (grams)	Calories
Chestnuts (¼ cup)	36	0	0	5	tr	7	2	tr	134
Filberts, hazelnuts (¼ cup)	34	tr	23	tr	8	3	21	2	213
Macadamia (¼ cup)	34	0	0	0	0	2	25	4	235
Mixed nuts with peanuts (¼ cup)	36	tr	7	tr	4	3	20	3	219
Peanuts (¼ cup)	36	0	0	0	3	3	18	2	209
Pecans (¼ cup)	27	tr	35	1	1	2	18	2	180
Pistachios (¼ cup)	32	tr	75	2	1	3	15	2	185
Walnuts (¼ cup)	25	tr	31	1	1	1	15	1	161

Food Description/ Portion	Weight (grams)	Beta Carotene (mg)	Vitamin A (I.U.)	Vitamin C (mg)	Vitamin E (mg)	Dietary Fiber (grams)	Total Fat (grams)	Saturated Fat (grams)	Calories
SEEDS									
Pumpkin seeds (¼ cup)	35	tr	131	1	1	2	15	3	180
Sesame seeds (¼ cup)	32	tr	21	0	1	3	18	2	188
Sunflower seeds, hulled (¼ cup)	36	tr	18	1	18	2	18	2	205
SALAD DRESSINGS									
Blue cheese, commercial (2 Tbs.)	31	tr	64	1	3	tr	16	3	154
Blue cheese, low calorie (2 Tbs.)	31	tr	24	1	tr	tr	tr	tr	6
French, commercial (2 Tbs.)	31	tr	21	0	2	tr	13	3	134
French, low calorie (2 Tbs.)	33	tr	529	0	0	tr	tr	0	3

Food Description/ Portion	Weight (grams)	Beta Carotene (mg)	Vitamin A (I.U.)	Vitamin C (mg)	Vitamin E (mg)	Dietary Fiber (grams)	Total Fat (grams)	Saturated Fat (grams)	Calories
Italian, commercial (2 Tbs.)	30	tr	23	0	2	tr	14	2	137
Italian, low calorie (2 Tbs.)	30	0	0	0	1	tr	3	tr	32
Mayonnaise, commercial (2 Tbs.)	28	tr	77	0	6	0	22	2	198
Mayonnaise, type 27% fat (2 Tbs.)	28	0	0	0	1	0	8	1	85
Mayonnaise, imitation (2 Tbs.)	30	tr	36	0	1	0	6	1	69
OTHER FATS									
Butter, stick (1 tsp.)	5	tr	145	0	tr	0	4	2	34
Butter, whipped (1 tsp.)	3	tr	92	0	tr	0	2	2	22

Food Description/ Portion	Weight (grams)	Beta Carotene (mg)	Vitamin A (I.U.)	Vitamin C (mg)	Vitamin E (mg)	Dietary Fiber (grams)	Total Fat (grams)	Saturated Fat (grams)	Calories
Coconut, shredded, unsweetened (1 tsp.)	2	0	0	tr	0	tr	1	1	11
Olives, black, ripe (3 medium)	12	tr	48	tr	tr	tr	1	tr	14
Olives, green, plain, stuffed (3 medium)	12	tr	36	0	tr	tr	2	tr	14
Peanut butter, creamy (2 Tbs.)	32	0	0	0	3	2	16	3	188
Shortening, animal/vegetable (1 Tbs.)	13	0	0	0	1	0	13	5	115
SNACK FOODS AND DESSERTS									
SNACKS									
Corn chips (1 cup)	26	tr	73	0	1	1	9	1	138

Food Description/ Portion	Weight (grams)	Beta Carotene (mg)	Vitamin A (I.U.)	Vitamin C (mg)	Vitamin E (mg)	Dietary Fiber (grams)	Total Fat (grams)	Saturated Fat (grams)	Calories
Popcorn, homemade with fat (1 cup)	11	0	0	0	tr	1	2	2	52
Popcorn, no fat/salt (1 cup)	8	0	0	0	tr	1	tr	tr	31
Potato chips (1 cup)	27	tr	2	7	1	1	10	1	149
Pretzel, hard type (1 cup)	44	0	0	0	tr	2	2	tr	170
Rice cakes, plain (1 piece)	9	tr	8	0	tr	1	tr	tr	35
DESSERTS									
Angel food cake (1/12 cake)	53	0	0	0	0	tr	0	0	127
Brownie, chocolate, without nuts (1 bar)	30	tr	40	0	tr	1	5	2	120

Food Description/ Portion	Weight (grams)	Beta Carotene (mg)	Vitamin A (I.U.)	Vitamin C (mg)	Vitamin E (mg)	Dietary Fiber (grams)	Total Fat (grams)	Saturated Fat (grams)	Calories
Candy, fudge, chocolate, with nuts (1 ounce)	28	tr	12	tr	tr	tr	3	1	111
Carrot cake, homemade, without nuts (1/10 loaf)	54	1	2,030	tr	2	1	14	2	245
Cheese cake, cream without crust/topping (1 piece)	84	tr	815	0	tr	0	19	12	268
Doughnut, cake (1 medium)	42	tr	139	tr	tr	1	8	3	155
Pastry, danish (1 pastry)	41	tr	24	0	3	1	16	6	214
Pudding, chocolate, canned (½ cup)	135	tr	203	1	1	1	7	1	203
Pudding, tapioca (½ cup)	100	tr	208	1	tr	tr	4	2	125

Food Description/ Portion	Weight (grams)	Beta Carotene (mg)	Vitamin A (I.U.)	Vitamin C (mg)	Vitamin E (mg)	Dietary Fiber (grams)	Total Fat (grams)	Saturated Fat (grams)	Calories
SUGARS AND SWEETENERS									
Honey (1 tsp.)	7	0	0	tr	0	0	0	0	21
Jam/Jelly (1 tsp.)	7	tr	1	tr	tr	tr	tr	0	18
Molasses, light/medium (1 tsp.)	7	0	0	0	0	0	0	0	15
Sugar, brown (1 tsp.)	5	0	0	0	0	0	0	0	17
Sugar, white (1 tsp.)	4	0	0	0	0	0	0	0	15
Syrup, corn/maple flavored (1 tsp.)	7	0	0	0	0	0	0	0	20

GLOSSARY

Antioxidants are chemical substances that stop the un-controlled production of harmful free radicals in our bodies and help to protect our bodies' cells. Beta caro-tene, vitamin C, and vitamin E are all examples of antioxidants.

Beta carotene is partially converted into vitamin A in the body. It is an antioxidant that can be found in dark-green vegetables and some deep-yellow and orange vegetables and fruits.

Calories are units of measure used to calculate the amount of energy contained in foods.

Carbohydrates, classified as either *complex carbohydrates* (starches) or *simple carbohydrates* (sugars), provide energy for our bodies.

Cholesterol is a waxy, fatlike substance that is produced in the body and is also obtained from foods of animal origin. It is needed to produce certain hormones and to construct cells, but too much cholesterol in the body can contribute to heart disease.

Dietary fiber is the nondigestible portion of plants.

—*Insoluble fiber,* which does not dissolve in water, helps to increase bulk and aid in regularity. It can be found in whole grains and brans of wheat, rye, and rice, vegetables, and fruits with edible seeds (e.g., strawberries).

—*Soluble fiber* dissolves in water and can help lower blood cholesterol. Sources include fruits, some vegetables, dried beans, pease, oats, barley, psyllium, and supplements.

Fat, a concentrated source of energy, carries certain vitamins. It also helps form cell membranes and supplies essential fatty acids, which the body cannot make itself.

—*Monounsaturated fats* may help lower blood cholesterol levels. They are found in such foods as peanuts, peanut oil, canola oil, olives, olive oil, and avocadoes.

—*Polyunsaturated fats,* found in liquid vegetable oils, tend to lower the level of cholesterol in the blood. Common sources include corn, safflower, soybean, and sunflower seed oils.

—*Saturated fats* are fats that harden at room temperature and tend to raise blood cholesterol levels. They are found in most animal and some vegetable products (e.g., butter, cream, whole milk products, coconut oil, palm oil).

Free radicals are chemical substances normally produced by our bodies, but which, when not blocked by antioxidants, can reproduce uncontrollably and cause harm to body cells.

International Unit is a standard unit of measurement common to some vitamin supplements, for example vitamin A, and is usually abbreviated as *I.U.* on vitamin supplement labels.

Minerals are inorganic (do not contain carbon) dietary elements that are necessary for health. They are essential for strong bones and teeth, blood formation, and clotting. Minerals also help regulate body functions and fluid balance.

Proteins are compounds made up of chains of amino acids. They provide structural support in our bodies and are a source of energy. The most complete sources of protein are found in dairy products and in meat, fish, and poultry.

Recommended Dietary Allowances (RDA) are recommended intakes of nutrients intended to meet most healthy peoples' needs for specified vitamins and minerals.

U.S. Recommended Daily Allowance (U.S. RDA) is established by the Food and Drug Administration (FDA) and is used to provide nutrient information on food and nutrition supplement labels. The U.S. RDAs express the food's nutrient value as a percentage of recommended levels and are a little higher than the RDAs in order to represent the nutrient needs of all healthy adults.

Vitamins are organic (carbon-containing) substances required in small amounts for the normal functioning of the body. They are necessary for growth and maintaining life. Along with minerals, vitamins are necessary for our bodies to utilize the carbohydrates, protein, and fat in the foods that we eat. Vitamins can be classified into two groups: fat-soluble and water-soluble.

—*Fat-soluble vitamins* are found in the fat portion of body cells and include vitamins A, D, E, and K.

—*Water-soluble vitamins* are found in the water portion of body cells and include the B vitamins and vitamin C.

REFERENCES

1. PREVENTING DISEASE: THE DIET CONNECTION

The American Heart Association Diet: An Eating Plan for Healthy Americans. American Heart Association, 1991.

Diet, Nutrition & Cancer: A Guide to Food Choices. U.S. Department of Health and Human Services with the National Cancer Institute. NIH Publication no. 87-2878, May 1987.

Eating Smart. American Cancer Society, no. 2042, March 1989.

Monthly Vital Statistics. National Center for Health Statistics, vol. 39, no. 13, August 28, 1991.

Nutrition and Your Health: Dietary Guidelines for Americans. U.S. Department of Agriculture and U.S. Department of Health and Human Services, Home and Garden Bulletin no. 232, 3rd ed., 1990.

The Surgeon General's Report on Nutrition and Health—Summary and Recommendations. U.S. Department of Health and Human Services, DHHS (PHS) Publication no. 88-50211, 1988.

An Ounce of Prevention

Block, G. "Dietary Guidelines & the Results of Food Consumption Surveys." *Am J Clin Nutr* 1991; 53:356S-7S.

Diet, Nutrition & Cancer: A Guide to Food Choices. U.S. Department of Health and Human Services with the National Cancer Institute, NIH Publication no. 87-2878, May 1987.

1991 Heart and Stroke Facts. American Heart Association, National Center, Dallas, Texas.

Antioxidants

Myeroff, W. "Winning A-C-E's." *Weight Watchers Magazine.* April 1991, pp. 22–24.

Okezie, I. A., et al. "Oxygen Free Radicals and Human Diseases." *J Roy Soc Health* 111 (5); October 1991, pp. 172–77.

Tolonen, M. *Vitamins and Minerals in Health and Nutrition.* New York: Ellis Horwood, 1990.

Toufexis, A. "The New Scoop on Vitamins." *Time,* April 6, 1992, pp. 54–59.

Watson, R. R., and Leonard, T. K. "Selenium and Vitamins A, E, and C: Nutrients with Cancer Prevention Properties." *JADA,* vol. 86, no. 4, 1986.

Vitamin A and Beta Carotene

Bakoulis, G. "Cancer Prevention?" *Health.* December 1987, pp. 57–58, 59, 65.

Bertram, J. S., et al. *Cancer Res* 1987; 47(11):3012–31.

Bjelke, E., et al. "Dietary Vitamin A and Human Lung Cancer." *Int J Cancer* 1975; 15:561–65.

Colditz, G. A., et al. *Arch Intern Med* 1987; 147:157–60.

Colditz, G. A., et al. "Increased Green and Yellow Vegetable Intake and Lowered Cancer Deaths in an Elderly Population." *Am J Clin Nutr* 1985; 41:32–36.

"Dietary Intake of Carotenes and the Carotene Gap." *Clinical Nutr* May–June 1988.

Friend, T. "Beta Carotene Cuts Heart Risk." *USA Today,* Nov. 14, 1991.

Gaby, S. K., Bendich, A., Singh, V. N., and Machlin, L. J. *Vitamin Intake and Health.* New York: Marcel Dekker, 1991.

Hirayama, T., et al. "Diet and Cancer." *Nutr Cancer* 1979; 1:67–81.

Peto, R., et al. *Nature,* 1981; 290:201–208.

Shekelle, R. B., et al. "Dietary Vitamin A and Risk of Cancer in the Western Electric Study." *Lancet* 1981; 2:1185–90.

Tolonen, M. *Vitamins and Minerals in Health and Nutrition.* New York: Ellis Horwood, 1990.

Toufexis, A. "The New Scoop on Vitamins." *Time,* April 6, 1992, pp. 54–59.

"Vitamin A Basics." The Vitamin Information Centre, Hoffmann-La Roche Ltd., Don Mills, Ontario, 1988.

Ziegler, R. G. "Vegetables, Fruits and Carotenoids and the Risk of Cancer." *Am J Clin Nutr* 1991; 53:251S–259S.

Vitamin C

American Journal Epidemiology, 1991, pp. 134–38.

Bayer, W., and Schmidt, K. "Vitamin C in Human Health." Vitamin Information Status Paper, F. Hoffmann-La Roche Ltd., Basel, Switzerland, 1990.

"Beyond Deficiency." New York Academy of Sciences Conference, Washington, D.C., February 10–12, 1992.

Eating Smart. American Cancer Society, no. 2042, March 1989.

Enstrom, J. E., Kanim, L. E., and Klein, M. E. "Vitamin C Intake and Mortality Among a Sample of the United States Population." *Epidemiology 3* May 1992, (3):194–202.

Gaby, S. K., Bendich, A., Singh, V. N., and Machlin, L. J. *Vitamin Intake and Health.* New York: Marcel Dekker, 1991.

Howkins, M. A. "The Nutrient Gap." *Glamour,* April 1992.

Jacobs, M. M. *Vitamins and Minerals in the Prevention and Treatment of Cancer.* Boca Raton: CRC Press, 1991.

Scherb, K. "A New Take on Vitamin C." *Weight Watchers Magazine,* February 1992, pp. 20–23.

Tolonen, M. *Vitamins and Minerals in Health and Nutrition.* New York: Ellis Horwood, 1990.

"Vitamins for Vision." *Healthy Food: Supplement to the Journal of the American Dietetic Association,* Autumn 1991, p. 9.

"Vitamin C Found to Serve as Antihistamine." *Food Chemical News* vol. 33, no. 10, May 6, 1991.

Vitamin E

Chan, A., et al. "Differential Effects of Dietary Vitamin E and Antioxidants on Eicosanoid Synthesis in Young Rabbits." *J Nutr* 113:813–819, 1983.

Howkins, M. A. "The Nutrient Gap." *Glamour,* April 1992.

Jacobs, M. M. *Vitamins and Minerals in the Prevention and Treatment of Cancer.* Boca Raton: CRC Press, 1991. Preface.

Knekt, P. "Vitamin E and Cancer Prevention." *Am J Clin Nutr* 1991; 53:283S-6S.

Riemersma, R. D., et al. "Risk of Angina Pectoris and Plasma Concentration of Vitamins A, C, and E and Carotene." *Lancet* 337 (8732), January 5, 1991, pp. 1–5.

Tolonen, M. *Vitamins and Minerals in Health and Nutrition.* New York: Ellis Horwood, 1990.

"Vitamin E Lives Up to Its Image as Protective Nutrient." *Environmental Nutrition* vol. 12, no. 1, January 1989.

"Vitamins for Vision." *Healthy Food: Supplement to the Journal of the American Dietetic Association,* Autumn 1991, p. 9.

Do You Need to Take a Vitamin Supplement?

Gaby, S. K., Bendich, A., Singh, V. N., and Machlin, L. J. *Vitamin Intake and Health.* New York: Marcel Dekker, 1991.

"The Supplement Story: Can Vitamins Help?" *Consumer Reports,* January 1992, pp. 12–13.

The Facts on Fiber and Fat

Dietary Fiber

Eat Right. American Cancer Society, no. 2099, 1988.

"NCI Urges Dietary Guidance on Benefits of High-Fiber Diets." *Food Chemical News* November 25, 1991, p. 75.

Waldholz, M. "High-Fiber, Low-Fat Diet Helps Prevent Cancer of Colon and Rectum, Study Says." *Wall Street Journal,* January 15, 1992.

Cruciferous Vegetables

Diet, Nutrition & Cancer Prevention: A Guide to Food Choices. U.S. Department of Health and Human Services and National Cancer Institute, NIH Publication no. 85-2711, July 1985.

Hattner, J. A. "Anti-Cancer Chemical Identified in Broccoli," *Issues In Food Safety,* vol. 5, issue 1, May 1992.

Cholesterol and Fats

Diet, Nutrition & Cancer Prevention: The Good News. U.S. Department of Health and Human Services, NIH Publication no. 87-2878, September 1987.

Eat Right. American Cancer Society, No. 2099, 1988.

Liebman, B. "Clues to Colon Cancer." *Nutrition Action Healthletter* March 1990.

"Lipids and Cancer." CRN report on FDA food labeling proposal.

Nutrition and Your Health: Dietary Guidelines for Americans. U.S. Department of Agriculture and U.S. Department of Health and Human Services, Home and Garden Bulletin no. 232, 3rd ed., 1990.

2. SELECTING AND PREPARING FOODS

Reducing Nutrient Loss

Corbin, C. *Nutrition.* New York: Holt, Rinehart and Winston, 1980.

Selected Cooking Methods

Diet, Nutrition & Cancer Prevention: A Guide to Food Choices. U.S. Department of Health and Human Services and National Cancer Institute, NIH Publication no. 85-2711, July 1985.

Hellmich, N. "Reducing Cancer Risk of Grilling," *USA Today,* May 30, 1991, p. 4D.

3. EXPERT ADVICE

The American Heart Association Diet: An Eating Plan for Healthy Americans. American Heart Association, 1991.

Eating Smart. American Cancer Society, no. 2042, March 1989.

Nutrition and Your Health: Dietary Guidelines for Americans. U.S. Department of Agriculture and U.S. Department of Health and Human Services, Home and Garden Bulletin no. 232, 3rd ed., 1990.

Recommended Dietary Allowances. National Research Council, National Academy of Sciences, 10th ed., 1989.

Sodium, Think About It . . . U.S. Department of Agriculture and Department of Health and Human Services, Home and Garden Bulletin no. 237, May 1982.

4. HOW TO USE THIS GUIDE

The Lowdown on Food Labels

Watson, R. R., and Leonard, T. K. "Selenium and Vitamins A, E, and C: Nutrients with Cancer Prevention Properties." *JADA* 1986, vol. 86, no. 4.

5. FOOD TABLES

Nutrient values in this book are derived from the University of Minnesota Nutrition Coordinating Center's (NCC) Nutrient Database Version 20, release date October, 1991.